When Movement Hurts.

A Self Help Manual for Treating Trigger Points

Barbara J. Headley, MS, PT

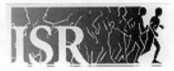

Innovative Systems for Rehabilitation
Boulder CO

This publication is designed to provide accurate and authoritative information in regard to the subject matter covered. It is sold with the understanding that neither the author nor the publisher are engaged in rendering professional services to the readers of this text. If legal, accounting, medical, psychological or any other expert assistance is required, the services of a competent professional person should be sought. ADAPTED FROM A DECLARATION OF PRINCIPLES OF A JOINT COMMITTEE OF THE AMERICAN BAR ASSOCIATION AND PUBLISHERS.

This book is not as complete and thorough as the Myofascial Pain and Dysfunction. The Trigger Point Manual, Vol 1&2. It is important that health professionals, in assisting clients with treatment of myofascial trigger points, refer to the reference list if they are not familiar with these manuals.

Library of Congress Catalog Card Number: 96-95018

ISBN #: 0-929538-14-5

To obtain copies of When Movement Hurts, contact:

OPTP
P.O. Box 47009
Minneapolis MN 55447-0009
612/553-0452
800/367-7393

This book is dedicated to David Simons, MD who, in partnership with Janet Travell MD, researched and wrote the definitive work on myofascial trigger points. David's commitment to document the movement dysfunction resulting from having myofascial trigger points has focused much of my clinical research and writing. He has shared his time, his enthusiasm and his wisdom with me, for which I am indebted.

As co-author of the two volumes of Myofascial Pain and Dysfunction: The Trigger Point Manual, it has been increasingly clear to me that there is an urgent need for a book like When Movement Hurts. We must all be grateful to Barbara Headley for fulfilling this need so well.

Barbara is uniquely suited to be the author. On one hand, she speaks with the authority of a patient who has been through the suffering and, on the other hand, with that of a physical therapist, a professional who understands the answers, and who is a pioneer in opening up new frontiers of our understanding of myofascial trigger points (TrPs).

She suffered a work-related back injury and became another victim of the worker's compensation medical "care" system. Since she suffered musculoskeletal pain that was caused largely by TrPs, and since the TrPs do not show up on x-rays or in lab tests, Barbara was quickly labelled as one of those worker's compensation patients who exaggerate their pain for the sake of increased compensation. Many patients are forced into this role because of the lack of understanding as to the source of their pain by the health care professionals responsible for their care. This role is rarely their first choice. Above all, these patients, like Barbara, want nothing more than to get rid of the pain and return to their previous lifestyle. Labels such as "symptom magnifier" often delay diagnostic workup. More than five years after her injury, Barbara had surgery to remove floating disc fragments. Then, the battle against musculoskeletal pain resumed, and traditional physical therapy was of little benefit. Because of her remarkable perseverance and unusual resourcefulness, she paid close attention to what helped and what didn't, combed the literature and her past professional experiences until she realized that her muscles had myofascial TrPs that were responsible for much of her pain. She began to find answers.

As Barbara learned how to control her pain and recover her activity tolerance, she soon found that there were many others who had problems similar to hers. They also were victims of the lack of understanding by health professionals. This is understandable. Few practitioners today have received training in the considerable palpation skills necessary to effectively diagnose the presence of TrPs. Many practitioners use techniques that can provide effective treatment of TrPs. However, they often don't understand that it is the TrPs that they are treating and so apply the treatment with reduced or no effectiveness, because of lack of training.

Unfortunately, at this time, you the patient must become sufficiently educated as to what TrPs are, how one diagnoses them, and what treatment approaches are most effective so that you can decide for yourself which self-proclaimed myofascial pain experts know enough to resolve the TrP component of your pain. This book provides invaluable guidelines for helping you to make that critically important decision.

Throughout this book, Barbara occasionally makes passing reference to her personal experiences. These references assure you, the reader, that this authoritative book offers an understanding and deep appreciation of your frustrations and hopes with practical descriptions of what the problem is and what you can do about it. This book shows you a way to regain control of your pain and your life so that you can call the shots and not have the pain calling them for you.

David Simons, M.D.

Acknowledgements

This book could not have been written had it not been for an orthopedic surgeon willing to look beyond the labels imposed on me by the workers' compensation system. I will be forever grateful to Tom Rieser, MD for listening to me. After six years, my life moved on and I sought to catch up with the rest of the world.

Through a new speciality in physical therapy, the many patients I have seen have refused to let me quit, take the easy way out, and I am indebted to them for reminding me as a professional that it is my job to look beyond the labels and the obvious. Each patient has added to my understanding of myofascial pain syndrome as a movement disorder.

Dr. David Simons has been, for four years, a personal mentor and motivator, always encouraging me to prove my assumptions and clarify my treatment approaches. I have completed endless hours of clinical research projects thanks to David's gentle pushing.

I have had two silent partners for the last ten years. My father's memories remind me of the importance of education and the written word. From my mother, there was money for the first sEMG equipment with which to begin this quest and encouragement to act on my dream.

I must thank the artist, Paulette Livers Lambert for her design of the book's cover, and the photographs on the front cover from David Lissy. For the remaining photos I am indebted to Kelly Madigan, Kirsten Treuman, Ambryn Headley, Jim Veraldi and Jennifer Headley for enduring numerous photo sessions and helping me bring this book to its illustrated format. Editing and proof-reading was done by Cheryl Riegger-Krugh, ScD, PT, Assistant Professor in the Physical Therapy Program at the University of Colorado Health Sciences Center, Denver CO. I am most grateful for her comments and assistance.

The journey that brought me to this book began in 1983 with a back injury. Struggling to validate my low back pain for five years in workers' compensation, I kept company with a journal after friends stopped calling. After five and a half years of being told the pain was "all in my head" a surgeon identified two central disc herniations and multiple disc fragments. The day after surgery the crushing pain was gone; but my journey was far from over.

My body no longer knew how to move without pain and dysfunction. Rather than "learning to live with the musculoskeletal pain" I fought back, exploring movement and discovering the phenomenon of myofascial trigger points. From the moment I deactivated my first trigger point I was able to begin to alter my own movement dysfunction and normalize the way I moved. The musculoskeletal pain was not only manageable, but I learned that if I kept the trigger points under control I could be painfree and very active. My training as a physical therapist enabled me to chart a new course in exploring movement dysfunction. Considered unemployable, I opened a clinic so I could work. The "failures" in workers' compensation were sent to the clinic and my work of documenting myofascial and movement dysfunction began in earnest. Using the technology of surface EMG I have sought to understand WHY patients fail and to offer them a new course of action.

My own journey is a gift not only to myself, allowing me to work with mentors such as Dr. Simons, but for the hundreds of patients that have come to me, seeking answers and willing to alter their own journey. They reinforce daily the value of a sense of control, inner skills and effective change. One of many poems I have written as a patient appears on the next page.

Barbara J. Headley, MS PT

Figure 1

3 a.m.

I fear most
    awakening at 3 a.m.;
    for it is then. . .

        that I am totally alone
        with myself
        and with my pain. . .

        Feeling that no one cares,
        and if they do,
        they cannot help. . .

        I lay awake with a sense of dread,
        a foreboding that tomorrow
        brings only more of the same. . .

        I tremble, feeling trapped,
        fearing the demons of my sleep,
        the nightmare that surrounds me. . .

        I seek security, reassurance
        that, somehow, things will change
        tomorrow. . . someday. . .

        I feel betrayed by my body, threatened,
        for I cannot run
        from the pain within.

In my world, with its pain,
    it is always "3 a.m."

bj headley
Copyright 1986, when pain had controlled my life for 3 years

Table of Contents

Figures

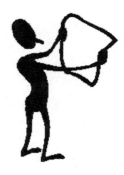

It is only after we have conquered

adversity that we label it a challenge.

-bj's soul scraps

Chapter 1

Symptom Management of Muscle Pain

The type of muscle pain that is due to trigger points, or knots in muscles, is generally referred to as "myofascial pain syndrome." The term myofascial pain syndrome (MPS) is often used generically, referring to muscle pain that might not be specific to myofascial trigger points (TrPs). There are many other terms for painful muscle syndromes, some of which are synonymous, some referring to other disorders involving muscle. These terms may include fibrositis, fibromyositis, fibromyalgia, fascitis, myositis, myofascitis and muscular rheumatism. Myofascial TrPs are very common and are a major source of musculoskeletal pain and dysfunction.

Muscle pain is primarily related to myofascial pain syndrome and involves trigger points. These TrPs are areas in muscle that are hard and painful. They are found in nodular or long, ropey bands within the muscle. The exact location of the TrPs within any muscle is very consistent, as are the referred pain patterns which emerge from an active TrP. These patterns of referral allow professionals and patients to find and relieve the source of the problem rather than misguidedly treat only the area that hurts.

In this type of muscle pain the problem seldom originates where the pain is experienced. Like a detective, one must seek out where the problem comes from and address the cause, rather than treat only the symptoms. This book is written to help you understand TrPs, and to assist you in finding the source of your symptoms. This enables you to learn many of the skills necessary to manage your own symptoms.

The benefits of being able to treat your own muscle pain is obvious. The body retains the effects of old injuries and habits. As a result, the activities that we enjoy are often accompanied by muscle pain. Sports or hobbies begin to cause pain as may some job tasks. The ability to continue enjoying activities can center on the ability to manage the symptoms before they interfere with activity or life. I learned this through personal experience. This ability provides a freedom to be more active, traveling and engaging in new activities more easily.

I travel frequently all over North America and Europe. Upon arriving at my destination, I frequently must stand and lecture 8 to 10 hours. If I had to teach for several days after activating several TrPs during a long flight and carrying luggage, but did not know how to reduce the discomfort, I would not do the traveling that I enjoy and consider a necessary part of my work. I also enjoy golf, hiking, biking and cross county

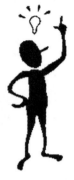

Figure 2

Who is in control ?
You or the pain.....

The following questions will help you determine the extent to which you may already function as a symptom manager.

1. When you are doing an activity you enjoy and begin to experience symptoms do you....
   a. stop the activity out of fear the pain will increase
   b. stop the activity temporarily, do something about the symptoms and return to your activity
2. How many activities have you stopped doing because the last few times you did them your symptoms increased, and you know that will happen again?
3. When friends call and want to go out, do you .....
   a. thank them but always refuse the invitation, knowing you would be sitting too long and would have more discomfort
   b. thank them and plan the outing so that you can cut it short if you need to without changing the others' plans
4. When you need to stay in a motel overnight, do you....
   a. dread the entire trip, knowing you won't sleep
   b. ask for a firm bed and make arrangements for a chair which will be comfortable.

skiing in spite of my back surgery. I have learned that in order to enjoy these activities and not have to limit my activities for days afterward, I must treat the muscle pain <u>before</u> it limits my function. Self management skills such as the ones I have learned allow anyone to be more active. I view the pain as something I can challenge and by adapting, I can extend the edge of my limitations without risking harm.

Imagine being able to play tennis on an occasional weekend and not being sore for days or painting a room as a surprise for a family member, knowing you will be able to immediately address the muscles that are sore and overworked. Soreness related to muscle pain is not necessarily related to an old injury, muscle damage, or aging.

Flare Ups

These occasional flare-ups are considered by most of us as part of getting older and something that we have been told that we must learn to accept. Certainly there are changes our body undergoes as we age, but some of the discomfort I treat in elderly people can be reduced or easily managed. Arthritis is a problem that develops in the joints; the portion of someone's pain that arises directly from the joint may not be eliminated. However, people with arthritis often have pain from muscles that have learned to work harder due to TrPs, compensation and probably reflex factors. The pain from the muscles, with their TrPs, can be treated.

If you had persistent daily pain from arthritis and had the opportunity to reduce the pain by 50% would you be willing to spend 10-15 minutes a day doing the necessary self management? That pain reduction might enable you to enjoy your grandchildren, play a full game of golf, or keep up with your friends on a short biking trip. Problems like arthritis cannot be totally alleviated with muscle pain techniques, but the techniques can reduce the level of daily muscular pain experienced.

Self Management

With self management skills you do not have to wait for a week until you can get an appointment to see someone, nor do you always have to interrupt your busy schedule. Self management skills mean that you can immediately take care of the problem when it <u>begins</u> to flare up, reduce the effects of the pain on your level of function, and continue with what is enjoyable and important to you. You'll also know when you need the help of an experienced professional.

Another important component of managing your own muscle pain is that YOU have a sense of control over your symptoms. That sense of control is critical in understanding the difference between your feeling in control, versus your feeling the pain is in control. If you feel you are in control you will be more active, you will be more willing to take on new challenges, and you will be less dependent on health care professionals. The ability to address your symptoms as they develop, before they limit your activity, are significant factors in dealing with muscle pain.

This manual is designed to complement the treatment you receive from a health care provider and can assist in your learning necessary skills. It can assist in the program developed by a physical therapist, complement the soft tissue work done by a massage therapist, or serve as an adjunct to the medication program prescribed by your physician. For some, this manual may eliminate the weekend warrior discomforts and avoid medical intervention entirely. Remember - if the self management skills do not work relatively quickly, more problem solving with a health care professional may be necessary. A good problem-solver and self manager knows there are times to ask for help.

Muscle Pain

There are three key points in the management of muscle pain:

☒ Understand the mechanism of muscle pain
☒ Know the components to effective management of muscle pain
☒ Learn to problem solve symptoms and use the proper self management skills.

Each of these components will be dealt with in one of the following chapters.

How Does Pain Interfere with Activity?

Some common guidelines may be helpful in noting at how much your activity level might have changed due to persistent muscle pain. The following scales help to examine your pain now and to measure how that pain changes as you learn to use the tools in this book.

A. The Visual Analog Scale

One of the most common pain measurement tools is called a visual analog scale. Using the numbers 0-10, rate your pain. Zero means no pain, and 10 refers to pain so severe you would consider not only going to an emergency room, but committing suicide. Fillingl in the Visual Analog Scale assists in becoming more aware of the changes in your pain as you begin

Pain Visual Analog Scale

1___2___3___4___5___6___7___8___9___10

to develop some self management skills.

4

B. Pain Variation

These questions help you to recognize the changes in your pain. As you relate changes in your pain rating to activities you will have begun to recognize key elements in being a symptom manager. Use the 1-10 scale.

Rate your pain

at its worst:_____

at its best:_____

Rate your average pain:_____

Rate your pain

in the morning:_____

in afternoon:_____

in evening:_____

C. Pain Interference

This component helps you to see how your behavior and activity might be modified due to the pain. Think about the questions, and jot down your comments. Review your answers after you have used this manual.

How well do you sleep?

_____

_____

Do you feel rested in the morning?

_____

Activity Avoidance

What activities do you avoid?

1._____

2._____

3. _____

4._____

Figure 3

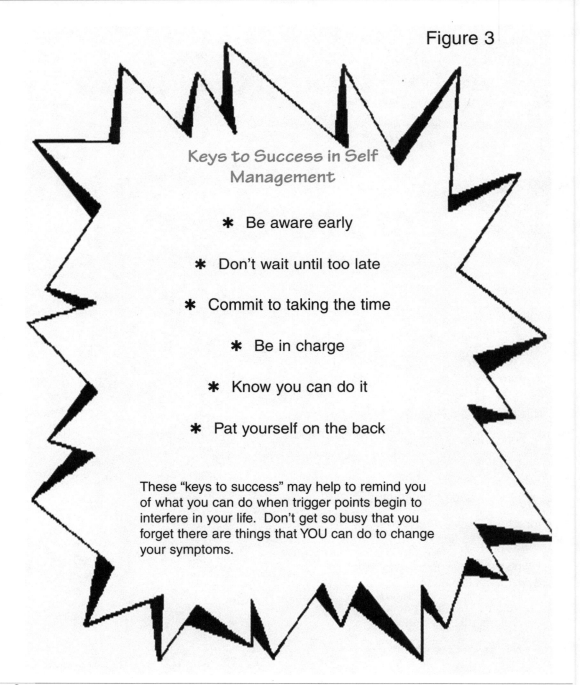

Keys to Success in Self Management

✻ Be aware early

✻ Don't wait until too late

✻ Commit to taking the time

✻ Be in charge

✻ Know you can do it

✻ Pat yourself on the back

These "keys to success" may help to remind you of what you can do when trigger points begin to interfere in your life. Don't get so busy that you forget there are things that YOU can do to change your symptoms.

Chapter 2

Mechanism of Muscle Pain

Muscle pain may arise from injury to the muscle fibers or the surrounding tissues. Muscle pain may involve the end of the muscle, where the muscle attaches to its tendon or bone, the tendon, or its membranes. Tearing of the muscle leads to muscle pain, as crushing or impact trauma leads to muscle bruising. Inflammation of the tissues surrounding the muscle fibers may also result in muscle pain.

Muscle pain may be related to sudden stretching of a tight muscle, sustained contraction, repetitive movement or unexpected strong contraction of the muscle for a heavy load. The pain may be related to extreme fatigue, cramping or spasm in the muscle. Many types of muscle pain appear to be related to by-products of muscle use that are not rapidly cleared. These by-products may cause irritation of pain-type nerve endings, signaling to the brain what we experience as pain. MPS from TrPs is only one form of muscle pain, and is the focus of this book. Some related readings can be found in Appendix C.

Figure 4

Factors that Activate Trigger Points:

1.) Chronic muscle strain

2) Repeated excessive muscle activity

3) Acute overload

4) Chilling of fatigued muscles

5) Nerve root compression

6) Anxiety tension states

Trigger Points

The muscle pain related to MPS and TrPs manifest itself as "knots" in the muscle. These knots or cord-like bands in muscle are painful when pressure is applied to them, when the muscle contracts strongly, or when the muscle is stretched. The ropey, cord-like bands often appear before TrPs develop. Some individuals appear to be more genetically likely to develop TrPs. Referred pain from TrPs often is a surprise to individuals when the pain originates from somewhere else; they often have no idea the cause of the pain is so distant. Detailed localization of the referral pattern arising with pressure on an active TrP is the best starting point for finding the TrP responsible for the pain.

TrPs develop when a muscle is overloaded or when the muscle is suddenly asked to perform a task beyond its ability. The action may be catching someone or something as it is falling, trying to recover from slipping on a floor or a patch of ice, or trying to lift something too large (and often unexpectedly heavy). TrPs may also develop when a muscle, or a portion of that muscle, is overtired and is forced to continue working.

These changes in movement cause other problems besides pain. If one compensates for a long enough period of time, there may be changes in the joints and ligaments resulting in additional symptoms. Muscles that harbor active TrPs resist being fully stretched. Attempts to fully stretch the muscle are painful until the TrP is treated. The muscle also may appear weak and it fatigues easily. Lack of endurance is a common feature in muscles with myofascial TrPs.

> To alleviate symptoms from TrPs, it is critical to find the source of the problem rather than to treat only symptoms.
>
> It is equally critical that the factors causing the TrPs be addressed and the factors perpetuating the TrPs be resolved.

The Referred Pain Patterns of TrPs

One of the principal characteristics of TrPs is the referral of symptoms to another part of the body. This referral of pain, or even numbness and tingling, makes the source of the problem harder to find. The most common complaint associated with TrPs is pain. The pain may be aching that is deep and penetrating, burning or numbing.

Numbness and tingling are other common sensations related to active TrPs and their referred symptoms. This means, for example, that the numbness you feel in some of your fingers may come from a TrP behind the shoulder or in the side of your neck. Some TrPs, far from their referred pain, may not hurt at all until pressure is applied to them. We call these latent TrPs because they are trouble waiting for a chance to happen.

The areas where an active TrP and its referred zone are located may feel hot and are-hypersensitive to pressure. Skin touch may not be affected. A hypersensitive TrP causes someone to jump when pressure is applied to the TrP, especially if the pain that results is not expected. A few TrPs may cause other, less typical symp-

Figure 5

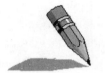

A Good Symptom Manager

The muscle pain related to TrPs can often be self managed and may only interfere with daily activity to a minor degree if the individual develops the tools of a good symptom manager.

1. Being a good symptom manager does not mean "pushing through the pain" and "ignoring it" no matter what.

2. A good symptom manager knows he/she can expect discomfort when they do certain activities.

3. They also know that they can limit the amount of pain by changing the way they perform activities, by stopping to stretch and give the muscles a break, and by treating the TrPs before they get out of control.

4. Being a good symptom manager means taking on the challenge of staying on top of the problem, and having good self management skills and taking control!

toms such as nausea, dizziness or sweating.

An acute TrP, limited to a single episode and muscle, may be easily resolved and may not recur. More commonly, however, the overloading of muscle occurs on an intermittent or regular basis, so that TrPs may become latent, or less active, but easily may be reactivated if the muscle becomes fatigued. Understanding what activates the recurrence of the TrPs becomes an important factor in controlling the problems that would otherwise limit function. The referral areas of TrPs may vary from those described in this manual. The more chronic the MPS, the more varied may be the referral patterns.

Trigger Points affect Movement

When a TrP develops in a muscle, it may change the way the muscle works. The muscle may shorten, putting abnormal tension and strain on other muscles, joints and ligaments. Muscles with TrPs may stop working. This shutdown may be global, i.e., the muscle is not working during any activities, or it may be selective, affecting only certain movements. If that muscle was primarily responsible for accomplishing the movement, other muscles that are not normally active have to accomplish the task.

When muscles take over for other muscles they are working as "second string" muscles, doing a job for which they are not optimally designed to do. These second string muscles

may fatigue more easily. They may also change the ease with which the joint moves through its range of motion as well as increase the stress on the joint. These changes in the movement of the primary muscle with the TrP, and its surrounding muscles and joints, may cause TrPs to develop in the second string muscles. This would result in pain developing in other areas, making the pain appear to move around. The sense that the pain is moving around is confusing to the individual with the TrPs and may also be confusing to the health professional seeing the individual as a patient. The patterns of referred pain and pain that seems to move around are two characteristics of referred muscle pain.

An example may help clarify the concept of muscle compensation. Let us assume that muscles "A,B,C" are those muscles that are used most often and most effectively to move the arm through a certain motion. If some or all of those muscles are not working, then muscles "K, L, M, P & Z" might be the muscles that are needed to continue performing the same task. The movement then involves more muscles, that are less able and less effective in performing the task, and apply more stress to both soft tissue and joint surfaces. More will be said about this in later chapters.

Figure 6

Trigger Points Change How We Move

The TrP affects the way we move. The change in how we move may be due to:

1.) the pain resulting from the TrP

2.) the inability of the muscle to move through its full length, stressing other tissues

3.) the muscle that is no longer doing its job

4.) another muscle taking responsibility for performing the activity

Chapter 3

Why Treating Muscle Pain is so Important

Of the many types of muscle pain, pain caused by TrPs may be one that you can handle without the assistance of a health care professional when the problem is not chronic. Acute muscle tears, strains or inflammation may require medical intervention. Do not overlook possible muscle damage by thinking that only TrPs cause muscle pain. You may consider consulting a physician or therapist before beginning to treat TrPs if you have had multiple injuries or have had pain for more than a few months. This manual is not a substitute for appropriate medical care.

Ignoring Trigger Points

The tendency is to ignore TrPs. After all, they are not life threatening, they seldom make it impossible to get around, and they don't hurt all the time. When a TrP is actively causing referred pain, it is also likely that muscle dysfunction is also present. After the acute phase of the pain settles down it is easy to ignore the TrPs. We need a reason to take time out of our busy lives. How often have we postponed a yearly physical exam or dental check up because we "don't have the time". Subtle muscle dysfunction is much like the tooth that is ignored until it becomes a more painful and more expensive problem.

An analogy might help. Some of those who own and drive cars check things like the air pressure in the tires regularly. Others choose not to do so. When the air gets low in one tire, the alignment of the car may suffer if the tire pressure is not promptly corrected. If the alignment

Figure 7

Active Trigger Points:

1.) may go away by themselves

2.) may persist but not cause other muscles to get sore

3.) can "spread" to other muscles, increasing symptoms, when other factors are present

of the car is finally compromised, it does not fix the problem to just fill the low tire with the correct amount of air. At that point, the complexity of the problem extends beyond the air in the tires. Both the air in the tires and the alignment must be corrected. So too, when TrPs are present over a long period of time, the postural alignment problems may become more extensive. Some tissues shorten, others lengthen, and these adaptive soft tissue changes must be addressed even if the TrPs have been treated.

A TrP in the low back, may shorten the quadratus lumborum muscle and result in the hip being hiked on the involved side. One leg is functionally shorter than the other. This is a bit like walking around with one high heeled shoe and one flat shoe. If you try walking like this for even a short period of time, you would develop pain in several locations, with increased pain if the leg length difference is present over a long period of time. There would be back pain, probably hip and sacroiliac joint pain, upper back pain and even headaches. If you were forced to walk like this for several months, removing the shoes so that you were then barefoot and level would not solve the problem. There would be muscles that had shortened, others that had lengthened,

joints that were inflamed and ligaments that were sprained. TrPs, although more subtle perhaps than this example, have the same effect on muscles, ligaments and joints.

Over the years, with old injuries and latent TrPs, there may be subtle, chronic changes in how you move. These movement changes may not cause you significant pain or even loss of function. You may not notice that you only play three sets of tennis before starting to get sore, rather than five. Then, some day, you acquire a new injury. With it, you find that you just don't recover as you should. You may then be a prime candidate for developing chronic pain. An ounce of prevention is your best insurance against chronic pain.

Releasing or treating the TrPs does not have to take a lot of time, but effective, early treatment can allow the tissue to restore its blood flow and allow the muscle to lengthen, restoring its normal resting length. Keeping the muscle healthy, and keeping it the proper length restores normal postural alignment and maximizes your chances of recovering fully from the next injury.

> Subtle trouble in movement may be a common sequelae of trigger points that hang around.

Find the Source of the Muscle Pain

Almost everyone has some form of muscle pain during their lifetime. For some, it may last

1-2 days, go away, and never return. For others, the pain is intermittent but bothersome, enough to limit activity on an occasional basis. For others, chronic pain may be present almost daily, nagging, wearing away one's energy and making it more difficult to have fun. Reaching into the medicine cabinet and taking some non-prescription medication may seem like a simple solution, but that only treats symptoms.

Treating the symptoms is common in our culture. Medication is one example. I was asked to see a physician at one of the clinics where I was teaching a course. He had had back surgery and by most standards was considered a "failed back." He felt he was managing fairly well with his symptoms, taking medication for the pain whenever it threatened to interfere with his daily schedule. He no longer performed surgery, but continued lecturing. His problem was relatively simple to evaluate. He had a slight leg length discrepancy which, after his back surgery, caused a low back muscle on one side (the quadratus lumborum) to develop TrPs and perpetuate his pain. Depending on his movements, he could get through some days, but had occasional days that were quite painful. His symptom management was simple - he killed the pain with medication.

> Movement disorder causes TrPs in other muscles, leading to muscle dysfunction as well as pain.

When shown how simple it was to treat the TrP and eliminate the cause of the pain he remarked: "This technique is almost as fast and as good as taking a pill." I would respectively beg to differ with him. By treating the TrP, he could eliminate the cause of the pain, rather than just the symptoms, which is all the pain medication can do. Furthermore, by treating the cause, which for him included adding a lift to his shoe, he also was reducing the chances of developing other problems that would develop from that primary site of muscle imbalance. By reducing the "domino effect" of other TrPs developing, he would feel better and raise his level of function over a long period of time. His medication, addressing only the symptoms, would necessitate continued use to mask the discomfort arising from secondary TrPs and compensatory muscle soreness. He had not yet fully grasped the idea that he could get rid of the problem, and avoid other secondary discomforts.

Reducing and Managing Flare Ups

By applying self management techniques as soon as the muscle pain begins to surface again, you can shorten the time your activity is limited by discomfort. When TrPs flare up, mus-

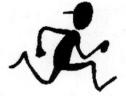

Figure 8

How determined are you to feel good?

1. Would you be willing to ask for a booth (or a table) and be willing to wait ten minutes for one if you knew you could then enjoy the meal?

2. Would you be willing to make a request for a hard mattress on a bed when you made your hotel reservations?

3. Would you also be willing to bring along a cushion to put in the car so driving was not painful?

4. How about walking all day - would you be willing to stop and stretch to take care of yourself?

5. You might be surprised at how many comments I get when I stop and take care of myself. Many others who are suf fering stop, but don't have good self management skills. They are impressed that someone can stop and take care of the symptoms.

cle activation is not well ordered, altering movement patterns.

Flare ups usually mean that a muscle has become overtired. Some muscles will be vulnerable to developing TrPs once you have had them. Be aware of when these muscles are getting tired and stop to stretch and normalize the muscle function. (See Chapter 4) A small pause in a busy day can avoid a lot of symptoms later. When the TrP becomes active again, the muscle may shut off, i.e., stop working. It is important to recognize that you are going to feel better, and stay more active, if the number of times the muscle becomes inhibited (stops recruiting) can be controlled. After you treat a TrP that has flared up, be aware of how you are moving, and focus on returning to normal. If you move in a dis-ordered fashion long enough, that movement pattern will begin to feel normal and "right."

The muscle dysfunction created by TrPs can create a vicious cycle of dis-ordered movement, as shown in Figure 9. When dis-ordered movement becomes a comfortable and safer habit, more effort is needed to return to efficient movement patterns.

Learning to Problem Solve

It is very common for individuals with chronic pain to determine that traveling is not something they enjoy any more due to the pain. Often trips are curtailed or eliminated. Many patients have told me that they are going on a trip to Disneyland, because they had promised the family years ago. They were already dreading the trip because they felt there were so many factors they could not change that would be painful for them.

The point here is that muscle pain can often

be controlled. You need to be a willing problem solver to be a symptom manager. While not every aspect of the trip can be changed, enough can so that you might be surprised at how much you might enjoy yourself. A key factor is to not resign yourself to the idea that, once you develop pain, you have to wait until you get home and make an appointment with someone to feel better, all the while suffering. Being a good symptom manager means learning how to take on the challenge of managing pain.

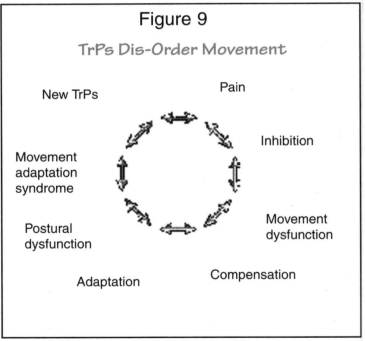

Figure 9

TrPs Dis-Order Movement

New TrPs

Pain

Inhibition

Movement adaptation syndrome

Movement dysfunction

Postural dysfunction

Compensation

Adaptation

Figure 10

Status of MPS and Fibromyalgia

CLINICAL PROBLEM	CHARACTERISTICS	HOW TO USE THIS MANUAL
1) Acute MPS Few TrPs	1 or several TrPs with specific onset. Resolves spontaneously or with brief treatment	Prompt attention to the TrPs should quickly relieve symptoms.
2) Chronic, complex MPS. Multiple TrPs active & latent	Multiple latent TrPs persist, & reactivate easily, contribute to muscle dysfunction & postural changes	This manual may be used initially in conjunction with a program designed by a health care professional.
3) Fibromyalgia	Tender points rather than TrPs, marked fatigue, poor endurance	Understand how to reduce loading on muscles using the Preventing Recurrence section
4) Fibromyalgia with TrPs	Generalized symptoms of fibromyalgia combined with localized MPS due to activity, fatigue or overuse	When MF TrPs activate, use the manual to reduce localized symptoms. Use Preventing Recurrence section to modify activity to prevent reactivation of TrPs

Chapter 4

Healthy Muscle Management

The ability to manage muscle pain is a skill you have already used, and one which you need only to refine. Everyone has had muscle pain in the past, and we have all taken the time to stop and rub the sore muscle. You instinctively do that for a reason. The pressure and deep massage you are exerting helps to loosen the tight, knotted tissue, restore blood flow and allow the muscle fibers to lengthen and relax.

This manual allows you to refine and develop the skills for healthy muscle management so that you can be even more effective. The tools described in this manual are not magic and should be considered one part of a complete program. These tools simply extend the reach of your arm and hand, or make it easier to

---

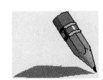

Figure 11

Healthy muscle management has several critical steps.

A. Identify the source
B. Apply pressure
C. Stretch
D. Relax
E. Be aware of subtle changes
F. Correct posture
G. Avoid mechanics that exacerbate

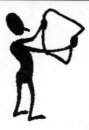

Figure 12

How TO:
Putting the Pressure on Trigger Points

1. Start with a moderate amount of pressure. You should feel some discomfort, and perhaps the referred pain pattern will become evident. Plan on holding that pressure for 10-12 seconds.

2. If the pressure increases the symptoms in those 10 seconds then the pressure is too much. You will need to get off the point, let it relax for a minute and then try again with less pressure.

3. When you are using the correct amount of pressure, the sense of how much pressure you are applying will decrease over the 10-12 seconds, even though you do not change how hard you are pushing. That change in the sensation of pressure is a partial release of the TrP.

4. You may then apply a very small amount more pressure and hold it for 10-12 seconds. You should get another release.

5. Repeat this procedure up to 4-5 times. The release may start to come more slowly. After the fourth time, let go and work on another point. In a few minutes you could go back and work on the same point again.

6. If you are pushing too hard, you will cause an increase in the symptoms; if you are pushing just enough, you will feel another release. If the TrP has been present for a long time it is unlikely you will get the knot to completely release in one session. Don't expect that to happen. It may not be until the next day that you experience the full benefit of treatment.

7. Keep the muscle lengthened to its full comfortable stretch length. This will greatly facilitate effectiveness.

8. Think about how long it took you to develop some of these TrPs; allow your body some time to adjust and relearn healthier muscle habits.

release TrPs that are located deep within several layers of muscle.

A. Identify the Source

Use this manual by looking through the pain patterns in the upper left corner of the pages that have pictures of TrP locations. These patterns may also be cross referenced by looking up common names for many syndromes in the index. For example, if you think of your pain as bicipital tendonitis, then you can look this up in the index and it will lead you to the TrP in the infraspinatus, a muscle in the back of the shoulder as well as other TrPs causing similar pain symptoms. The infraspinatus refers pain over the front of the shoulder joint. You could also find it by looking through the pages of shoulder joint pain and finding that the infraspinatus referral pattern looks like your pain referral pattern.

Treating the pain on the anterior side of the shoulder will not give you the relief you want. If the infraspinatus TrP is the pain generator, the source of the problem becomes the area that you treat. This may be a method of problem solving that seems very foreign. In fact, this is the same method that physicians have used to track gall bladder and heart attack problems to their source, allowing effective treatment intervention. The referral patterns in muscle have not been as well known, but they also have been used for years.

B. Pressure

When pressure is put on a TrP, the response is often one of "that hurts good", meaning that although it hurts, the pressure feels like just what you needed. Pressure, in fact, is one of the major components of treatment. However, too much pressure can result in the tissue springing back, the TrP getting tighter, and the pain increasing. "Just enough" pressure is the real key in working on TrPs. This policy of just enough applies whether you are using your finger, a friend's thumb or one of the tools you have found to be helpful.

If the TrP is very sensitive and you cannot tolerate pressure, you may need to desensitize it. This can be accomplished in a number of ways. You might use a vibrator, set to a very low setting and with a soft, facial attachment. Move the vibrator lightly back and forth across the area, spending more and more time directly over the TrP. Gradually, the TrP will tolerate more pressure and you can begin to apply the pressure directly.

If you work too hard on a muscle you may develop a bruise. Working too hard on the TrP also may make you sore for several days and indicates you are too aggressive. Treating TrPs is not a case where the "no pain, no gain" model is appropriate. Use a gentle model which will encourage the tissue to relax and tolerate the pressure. Deep tissue work, if needed, should be done by a skilled therapist.

Some people have waited so long for some method of controlling the pain they see this model of treatment as a "quick fix" to a very chronic problem. If you have only one or two acute TrPs, then you may effectively take care of them in just a few days. That is not the case with TrPs that have been present for a long time. You

Figure 13

Stretching for Health

1. Do the stretch slowly. The biggest problem with giving handouts to people without practicing the stretch with them first is that they do not understand where they should feel the stretch and if they are being effective. For that reason, many stretching programs have been abandoned and people have felt that they, or the stretching program, have failed.

2. As you are doing the stretch, you will reach a point where you begin to feel the tension in the muscle.

3. At this point, go only a little further. You want a nice, gentle stretch on the muscle, and you want to be able to hold that stretch for a minute. Not 10 seconds, not 30 seconds, but a full minute. Concentrate on relaxing the muscle being stretched. Relax slowly.

4. Don't bounce! Just go to the end range and hold it there. After a minute, if the muscle no longer pulls at that point, you may stretch a bit more while concentrating on not tightening up the muscle.

5. Don't try to stretch out fully in one day a muscle that has been tight for 10 years. If you don't stretch for several days, start again slowly.

6. After you have held the stretch for a minute, let it go.

7. You might gently massage the muscle again if you like.

8. You may repeat the stretch again several times, but each time you must hold the stretch for 60 seconds, and then release it slowly from the stretch position. This helps to release the knot after you have softened it, and will help that bundle of muscle fibers not tighten up as much after you stop working on it.

cannot change many TrPs and chronic problems in muscle tissue quickly. Respect that your body needs to make some other soft tissue changes as you release the TrPs. Give the tissue a chance to change in a fashion that you will have the best long term relief.

You can also work on the TrPs with massage. Tools such as the TAMM™ (Trigger point And Muscle Massage) Unit (used in the illustrations throughout this manul) will assist you in doing that to many of the body parts you find hard to reach. Again, start lightly and don't work so hard that you have to grit your teeth and tense other muscles. If the muscles around the area tighten up, then you are working too hard. Lighten up and find out what "just enough" pressure is. Using the roller for massage can be very helpful in loosening up and relaxing the entire muscle. Move along in the direction of the fibers (refer to the appropriate TrP page for a layout of each muscle). Work like you would roll out dough with a rolling pin, gradually increasing pressure. Do it for only a few minutes the first few times. You should not be more than mildly sore for more than two hours. Staying within these limits, you can gradually increase the length of time and the amount of pressure.

After working on the muscles, it is important that you provide the muscle with what it needs - water. Drinking plenty of water, may reduce soreness that often comes after treatment, and enhancing the ability of the tissue to recover its normal metabolism.

C. Stretch

The best time to stretch a muscle that has a TrP is right after you use pressure. This helps the knot to release even more, and will enhance the overall effect of the pressure techniques. A stretch has been included with each TrP, showing you where the muscle is located. This should help you determine if you are stretching the right muscle; it should feel like it pulls in that area. If you have another muscle that is tighter, limiting your ROM, you may feel it pull somewhere else. Then you might find that tighter muscle and work to stretch it out before returning to the muscle causing your pain.

If you only have the TrPs on one side, it is often helpful to stretch the other side as well. You will know how far the muscle should stretch and what it should feel like. Stretching the non-painful side will also help you compare changes in the shortened muscle with the normal side. If you try stretching the muscles without working on the TrPs with pressure first, the rest of the muscle may get longer, but the TrP may not change.

Changes take place all over the body when you start to change the length of muscles. Expect those changes to happen and don't worry about them. Your body has one fascial layer that reaches from head to toe and changes in one part of the fascia affect areas of the body remote from the initial injury. As you

feel a stretch, take a deep breath before going any further. Slowly exhale as you gently stretch the muscle. You might do this 3-4 times then hold the muscle in its lengthened position.

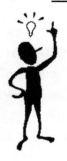

Reminders

1. Doing a stretch is also a good way to check to see if the muscle is getting tighter.

2. After the muscle and TrP have been released, you may find that you do not have to do all your stretches every day.

3. You may do some only a few times a week, then once a week.

4. If you are a good symptom manager, you may do the stretch only when you sense the muscle is getting tight, or the TrP is knotted up.

5. Any tightness in the muscle would be a signal to work on the TrP and resume the stretch again, if only for a few days.

6. A regular exercise program, with a stretching program, promotes healthy muscle habits.

You might consult with a therapist on occasion to give you some guidance and direction in working with your body. Helping your body to restore normal alignment (posture) and length in the muscles will help reduce future injuries. Postural dysfunction also brings with it subtle shifts in the joint alignment. These changes may be much less amenable to self management. When myofascial work does not result in the changes you expect, you may be missing some TrPs or you may need to look at joint alignment. Seek a therapist skilled in these areas for help.

restore normal length to a few muscles, other muscles will change their length to adapt to the new stresses, or reduction of stresses. This may cause discomfort that you might not be expecting in another area of the body.

Using your breathing you can help to increase the stretch to the muscle. When you have elongated the muscle enough to begin to

D. Relax

It is important when you are stretching the muscle that you relax it first. You do not want to be pulling against a tightly tensed muscle. Learn what it feels like to totally relax the muscle. Another technique that helps relax the muscle is to contract it first by taking the muscle to its most stretched position, and then contracting the muscle with a moderately strong contraction, but don't let the muscle shorten. Hold the contraction for 2-5 seconds, then let the muscle relax and try stretching it. You may be able to get a bit more length out of it. Do this 3-5 times if it helps. The contraction does not need to be very strong. The muscle will relax a bit more each time.

Some muscles, like the ones in the neck, tend to get tight when we are under stress, very tired or work at a desk If this is the part of the body you are working on, you must become aware of how tense you are holding the muscle, and remember to relax the muscles frequently during the day. Try relaxing and stretching the muscle each time you finish a phone call, or each time you stop at a red light.

E. Awareness

Correcting posture is very difficult for some of us. Part of the problem is that we have learned to stop listening to our bodies. As children, we squirmed when we began to get uncomfortable. We were told to sit still (and not listen any longer to the messages from within). In the early grades, a good student was one who could sit still and pay attention in class. Outside the classroom, reinforcement to ignore our bodies increased as we fell and scraped elbows or knees, as we began sports, and as we joined a workforce with its constraints on break times and freedom to move about.

Our culture emphasizes the model of "no pain, no gain" and "ignore the pain." Together, these and other messages often convince us that the pain is not anything we can change, so we work hard to put it out of our minds. When the pain is associated with something like arthritis, that message is reinforced. Arthritis is a disease of joints, and to some extent it cannot be eliminated (although medication can be used for the joint inflammation). When we are told arthritic pain is just part of getting old, there is an assumption that we are powerless to change it. In working with patients who have arthritis but who also have some muscle problems, the total picture of pain might be changed.

Addressing the symptoms related to muscles in individuals with arthritis might reduce the pain by 10 to 50 percent. Would some percentage reduction in pain be worth 20 minutes of your time each day to maintain? Many people feel somewhat amazed initially that they have some choice about their level of pain. In a few cases, patients have become mildly annoyed that they can choose between pain and control of their symptoms when they are in the midst of working or enjoying themselves, even when they know they will suffer if they ignore the early signs.

F. Correct Posture

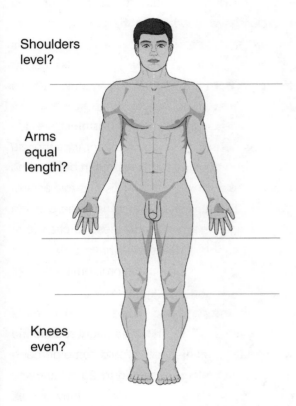

Shoulders level?

Arms equal length?

Knees even?

need some help to increase your awareness. You could start by using a mirror, or have a friend take some pictures of you standing and sitting so that you have something to look at objectively. You might notice that one shoulder is higher than another. You might also notice that your head is forward of your shoulders - it should be resting so that your ear is over your shoulde with the chin jutting forward. You might notice that one arm is turned in more than the other, or that one foot points out away from the

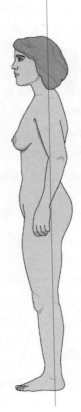

Is ear above shoulder?

Shoulder above hip?

Hip above ankle?

A down side of the "no pain, no gain", philosophy is that the individual typically will have little or no understanding of what increases or decreases their pain. They therefore have little control over it. Difficulty in being aware of one's body does not mean that you cannot work on your posture. It only means that you may

other foot more.

As you stand against a wall with your heels, buttocks, shoulders and head touching, you can note how much room there is between the wall and your lower back. Both lack of a space and too much space is a problem. This position may help you become aware of forward shoulders or head, tight hip flexors or an increased sway to your back.

Even lying on the floor can help you "see" your posture. As you lie on your back, notice where you are touching the floor. Note if the right and left legs touch in the same places with the same amount of weight. Where are your buttocks touching the floor? Is the weight the same on each side? What about your trunk - are both shoulder blades touching the floor in the same places with the same weight? Are both arms resting on the floor? Is one arm turned in more than the other? Are both shoulders in the same place in relation to the floor?

As you work on your TrPs you want to make sure that your posture enhances the gains you make on your TrPs. The cause and effect can become reversed. The forward head posture may first have been a result of some TrPs; now that posture could become the cause of the TrPs not going away. The better your posture, the easier it will be for the muscles to hold you up. Keep in mind that your head weighs as much as a bowling ball. Think how easy it might be to hold that bowling ball close to your body. Now imagine moving the ball several inches out in front of your body. The weight will tire your arms much more quickly. When your head moves forward from your shoulders, your neck muscles have to work very hard to not let it fall forward and drop down to your chest. That is what gravity is trying to do - get your head to fall farther forward. The muscles in the back of your neck and shoulders have to fight gravity all the time. That is a lot of work, and clearing TrPs in muscles working this hard is very difficult. Connecting postural habits with a strengthening program may exacerbate TrPs if they are not treated. Be careful when strengthening to not overly fatigue the muscles with TrPs and emphasize endurance rather than power.

F. Avoid mechanics that exaccerbate

Often the date and cause of an injury are very obvious. The TrP may have developed when playing tennis, carrying suitcases through an airport, or sitting in a car for hours. In many cases, the onset is more gradual and the cause not so easily identified. It may be up to you to find what caused the TrP to develop. With each TrP described in this manual are included some examples of how a TrP to become active.

If you learn that the TrPs tend to act up when you drive long distances, then you might take the time to get out of the car and stretch more often. You might also try stretching in the car, or having someone else take a turn driving. Finding out that you tend to develop TrPs while playing tennis, for example, does not mean that you have to stop playing. It may mean, though, that you will enjoy the game more if you stretch before playing and work to strengthen the muscles that are giving you the problem. If you have questions about the strengthening program consult a physical therapist, exercise physiologist or other knowledgeable professional.

If sitting at your desk and holding the phone with your shoulder is the problem, then you might have to look at how you can set up your desk differently, or use a headset. Finding the cause of the problem does not mean that activity must be avoided. It suggests only that you modify how you perform the activity.

On each TrP page there are suggestions about factors which may contribute to perpetuating each TrP. You may find other reasons unique to you, your job, or your sports. The more aware you are, the more you can control symptoms when they occur and determine how long they last.

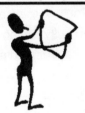

Figure 14

Self Management Tips using a Pressure Tool

Do's and Don'ts:

♦ Do use the tool sooner, rather than later. Having many trigger points to treat may mean that you might have intervened sooner.

♦ Stretch the muscle after using the tool for a better release.

♦ Stretch gently, don't bounce, hold for 30 seconds.

♦ Stretch often, for short periods of time, don't let the muscles get so tight or so fatigued.

♦ Even it it "hurts good", don't try to get rid of a chronic trigger point in one sitting.

♦ Do pay attention to your body; it knows when you need to get up and move around for a minute.

♦ Do exercise! It is the best prevention of musculoskeletal injuries, not to mention your spine, your cardiovascular system and your general health.

Self Management Tools

Tools for self management that are used to assist in treating TrPs are numerous and varied. Many pressure tools serve primarily to increase the length of one's reach or more easily allow pressure on an awkward-to-reach TrP. The TAMM™ Unit shown in this manual is only one of many tools. Others may focus on the application of direct pressure, such as the TheraCane® or Backnobber®. Others may make the massage to the muscle easier, i.e., the IntraCell®. Some TrPs can best be treated with tennis balls. Even the rolling pin has been found useful for TrPs in the arch of the foot!

The application of direct pressure to the TrP is as important as the stretching that should be done afterwards. Not only is gentle stretching advocated, but so is gentle application of pressure.

Some people find the pressure from plastic or wooden knobs too hard. Use of the TAMM Unit offers a variety of firmness in the ball attachments so that desensitization may occur and deeper pressure then tolerated. The pressure should focus on the area of the taut band that is sensitive; often a one half inch difference in location of the pressure decreases its effectiveness.

It is important in reducing postural dysfunction that the TrP be deactivated promptly.

Everyone would like to visit a massage therapist for any ache or pain, but many cannot. When traveling it is essential for me to decrease my symptoms promptly before postural dysfunction increases my pain and I am no longer comfortable to lecture, etc. These tools mean a sense of freedom for me that I otherwise cannot obtain.

Myofascial TrPs exist in a wide variety of patient populations. They may represent the primary pain symptoms, such as in failed low back pain, or a secondary pain complaint for a patient with arthritis. They may reflect our response to gravity's forces as we age and muscles have less postural holding power. Tools and self management may increase our ability to combat gravity's forces, allowing the freedom of higher activity levels and function as we age.

These tools should be part of a problem solving agenda not a replacement for medical diagnosis and treatment. Treatment of complex and chronic conditions may be enhanced by the use of these tools, but they may not replace the benefits of hands on care.

As managed care increases our challenge to be self managers, such tools as these increase our freedom from managed care's bureaucracy and limitations.

Figure 15

Each TrP page has been designed to offer you information about the trigger point and its symptoms on the left-hand page, the solution on the right-hand page. The following key is needed to understand the way the drawing has been done.

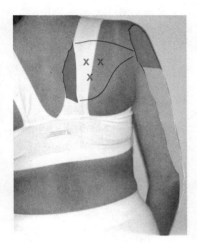

- The outline represents the borders of the muscle.
- The "X" indicates the locations of the TrPs.
- The dark red area is the area of primary pain.
  This may be in the same muscle or referred to another area.
- The light red areas or less common referral zones
- When the tool or stretch is shown, "X" indicate TrPs and the muscle is outlined

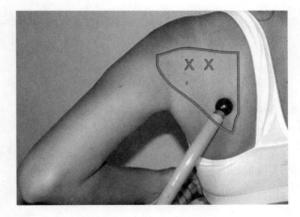

NOTE: Use descriptors as you shade in the body areas with your symptoms. You might want to identify one area as tingling, another as dull aching, another as sharp pain with motion.

Example:

Burning: xxxxxxxxx

Numbness: #########

Pins/needles: 0000000000000

Aching: ∧∧∧∧∧∧∧

Stabbing: ////////////////

Related Dx's: These are diagnoses that may represent similar pain problems.

Signs & Symptoms: Problems you may be experiencing.

Check these TrPs: Other TrPs that are often a problem when the one you are reading is active.

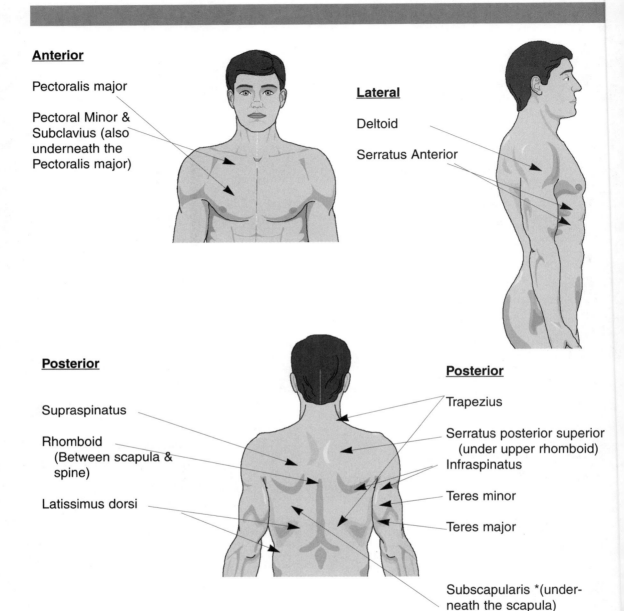

Anterior

Pectoralis major

Pectoral Minor &
Subclavius (also
underneath the
Pectoralis major)

Lateral

Deltoid

Serratus Anterior

Posterior

Supraspinatus

Rhomboid
(Between scapula &
spine)

Latissimus dorsi

Posterior

Trapezius

Serratus posterior superior
(under upper rhomboid)

Infraspinatus

Teres minor

Teres major

Subscapularis *(under-
neath the scapula)

Chapter 5

Shoulder & Shoulder Girdle Problems

Everyone has probably developed some sort of shoulder pain during their lifetime. The onset of the pain may be gradual and not related to any specific injury, or it may be sudden and very specific to a fall, a sporting activity, or a motor vehicle accident. The shoulder may only hurt at rest, or when using it, or perhaps when trying to sleep. The shoulder may feel like it "clicks" or gets "stuck" during one part of the arc of movement, or it may hurt mostly when you are just sitting quietly. Some shoulder pain is usually ignored by everyone. It may come, stay a few days, and leave. We may complain to someone, but the complaints are vague, and the pain cannot be pinpointed. With time, the shoulder pain may go away. But, sometimes it lingers.

Shoulder pain, like low back pain, can interfere with many daily activities. Most people take their body for granted; the free and painless use of a shoulder is no exception. The following body diagram for pain and checklist (p. 33) might be helpful for you to increase your awareness of when the symptoms come, where the symptoms are on the shoulder and then you can use this manual actively to do something to reduce the pain.

Not all shoulder pain is responsive to TrP work on the muscles. There is shoulder pathology that exists independent of muscle pain and may need to be addressed by other means. For those with muscular pain, the opportunity to do something about the pain, and increase your level of function, may be very beneficial. It will be helpful for you to become aware of where, when and how the shoulder pain develops or becomes a problem. Start with the body diagram below, then move on to the checklist.

Pain Diagram

One more opportunity for you to be more-aware is to fill in the pain drawing in the way that you would best describe the pain. The drawing on page 30 can be used, with symbols for the various types of discomfort you might be feeling. This will help you identify the discomfort in the

TrP drawings that follow. Remember, to understand how you can effectively manage your symptoms, you must have some awareness of when the symptoms change, and what occurs at that time.

NOTE: Use the descriptors from Figure 15, page 29 as you shade in the body areas with your symptoms. You might want to identify one area as tingling, another as dull aching, another as sharp pain with motion.

The Checklist:

1.] What time of day do you notice the pain the most?

2.] What activities make the pain worse?

3.] What activities make the pain better?

4.] What words would you use to describe the sensations? (for example, nagging, stabbing, annoying, sharp, dull ache)

5.] Is there a condition you can describe (for example, a rub, or a click)

6.] Does the problem occur only during one part of the range of shoulder movement?

7.] Do you avoid moving your arm in certain ways, to do certain things, because of the discomfort?

8.] Is your right shoulder level with the left shoulder, or is it higher, lower? Is the shoulder more forward than the uninvolved shoulder?

9.] When standing with your arms hanging down at your side, are both arms in the same position?

Often pain comes on suddenly. It may be after doing something as simple as brushing your teeth. You may wonder how such a simple task, that you have been doing most of your life, could cause so much pain. The chances are that the pain was caused by something you did prior to brushing your teeth, and that activity was simply the "straw that broke the camel's back". There is often a cumulative reason for pain that it is difficult for us to pin down because we have been doing the task without pain for years.

Common Minor Trauma

There are a number of problems that might arise slowly, not demanding our attention until the pain reaches a certain threshold or stops us from doing an activity that is important. When asking patients who have had chronic pain for years, they may say that no household chores increase their pain. But, when asking them which chores from a list might lead to an answer "Oh, I stopped doing those chores five years ago." Identifying these types of activities may also be very helpful in identifying the specific nature of the shoulder problems.

Pain may develop secondary to a problem identified as bursitis, tendonitis or impingement syndrome. Any of these diagnoses may warrant the attention of a physician or therapist. TrPs may exist along with these syndromes, and may be the reason why you are having some persistent complaints even after the primary problem has been treated. TrPs may mimic these syndromes, and looking for the active TrPs early may eliminate the need for some other medical care.

Acute Trauma

Acute trauma may result from a fall, from a sports injury or from unexpectedly catching a heavy object. Often, muscles prevent the joint from being injured. The soreness in the muscles after the injury may be TrP related, and are important to explore. If an acute injury necessitates surgery, the surgery may repair damage to joints or ligaments, but may not do anything for the muscles. Pain after an acute fall or after surgery is often related to the mis-use of muscles.

Cummulative Symptoms

A common and current problem now being reported is the pain and dysfunction that exists with poor posture or jobs that require sitting and prolonged static activity. Many health care providers are recognizing that there are biomechanical problems that often develop in the area of the shoulder blade and scapula that precede carpal tunnel syndrome. More about this in a later chapter.

Many injuries develop slowly, over time. These complaints may eventually lead to other biomechanical problems. If your posture includes rounded shoulders and a forward leaning head, you may have some TrPs to work on, and some muscles to strengthen.

Using this Section

TrPs seldom occur in only one muscle unless you have a minor problem and catch it early. For most people, by the time it becomes painful, there are several TrPs to work on. You will need, therefore, to identify one or more TrP patterns as representing your symptoms, and follow the recommendations about what other TrPs to look for in the pages that follow.

One more point. If you find that working on the TrPs alleviates your pain for only a short time, there may be other factors, such as a leg length difference, or postural problems that are making it difficult for you to get the TrPs under control. For these, you may need the assistance of a therapist to advise you and make recommendations.

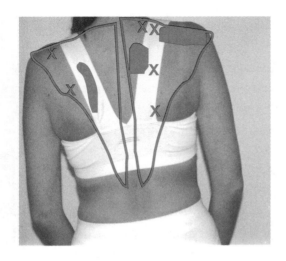

Related Dx's:

- Cervical pinched nerve
- Stiff neck
- Tension headache
- Temporomandibular joint disease

The Muscle:

The trapezius retracts the shoulder blade. The upper portion "shrugs" the shoulder. The upper and lower portions rotate the shoulder blade as you raise your arm.

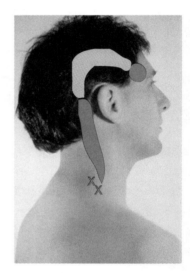

Signs & Symptoms:

- Severe neck pain at back of head
- Headache, often localized to temple or base of skull
- Burning pain along edge of shoulder blade near spine
- Sensitivity to heavy clothing on shoulders
- Brief episodes of dizziness or loss of balance
- Loss of ROM in neck

Causes:

- Acute: Fall
- Whiplash
- Chronic: Typing, especially with poor ergonomic design of workstations
- Static assembly work
- Compensatory posture
- Carry purse or book bag on one shoulder
- Upper arms that are short, not reaching arm rests
- Increase in pace, stress or fatigue
- Bra straps too narrow
- Prolonged desk work
- Round-shoulder posture
- Constant holding of shoulders up, as when under stress
- Holding arm up and forward for a long time

Refer to Index, Legend, Figures, Glossary & Abbreviations

Management Tips:

- This muscle lengthens as you tire, rounding the shoulders
- Shortening the muscle by brief contractions is more important than stretching it
- Stretch (below right) is done by grasping your hands in front of you and reaching as far as possible forward
- Use the upper trapezius stretch (below, center) to shorten the lower trapezius and counteract the rounded shoulders that develops with prolonged sitting

Preventing Recurrence:

- Correct work space
- Correct arm rest heights
- Stretch tight anterior chest muscles
- Reduce prolonged turning of head to one side, i.e., typing
- Carry purse tucked under arm or use fanny pack
- Carry backpack using both shoulder straps & slide shoulder straps to outside edges of shoulders
- Consciously relax muscles when stressed
- Replace foam with regular, firm pillow
- Strengthen to stabilize scapular muscles

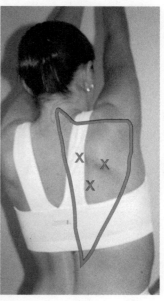

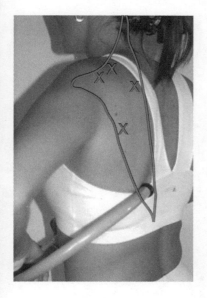

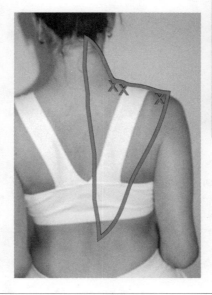

Check these TrPs:

Rhomboids
Supraspinatus
Levator Scapulae
Scalene

Remember the rules for stretching and applying pressure

35

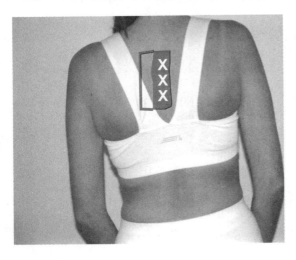

Related Dx's:

- Thoracic disc disease
- Cervical disc disease
- Thoracic sprain

The Muscle:

The rhomboid retracts the shoulder blade and rotates it so the shoulder joint turns downward as the shoulder blade comes closer to the spine

Signs & Symptoms:

- Pain along the border of the shoulder blade next to the spine
- Pain persists at rest
- Pain increases with motion
- Snapping and crunching noises may occur during movement of shoulder blade

Causes:

- Prolonged forward position of shoulder as when sitting at a desk
- Shortening in the pectoralis major
- Iliopathic scoliosis
- Carrying backpack or purse on one shoulder
- Atypical work position of arms overhead & back arched, i.e., painting ceilings
- Arm swinging while walking may cause pain once TrPs develop
- Chest surgery
- Leg length imbalance

Refer to Index, Legend, Figures, Glossary & Abbreviations

Management Tips:

- May use ball standing against wall or lying down, placing ball where "X" indicates TrP and symptoms are elicited
- When doing the stretch (below right) place your hands on the wall and then round your back, sliding your shoulder blades forward; this muscle is more often stretched than short ened. After the TrPs have been treated, strengthen the muscles bilaterally

Preventing Recurrence:

- Strengthen and shorten muscle by balancing it with length of pectoralis major to reduce forward shoulder posture
- Enhance stabilization of the shoulder blade
- Use of correct posture when sitting
- Ergonomic corrections if desk job is done
- Change arm positions on steering wheel when driving long distances
- Have good low back support when sitting

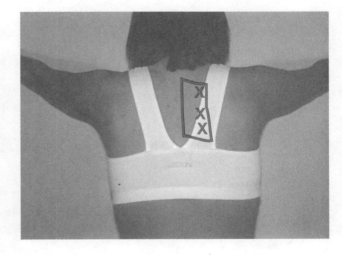

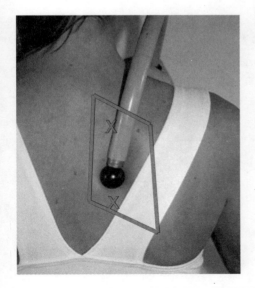

Check these TrPs:

Trapezius
Infraspinatus
Pectoralis major & minor

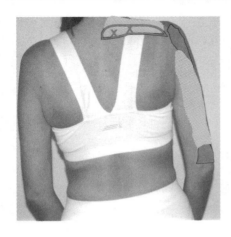

Related Dx's:

- Subdeltoid bursitis
- Cervical arthritis
- Bicipital tendonitis
- Bone spurs in cervical spine
- Rotator cuff tears

The Muscle:

The <u>supraspinatus</u> abducts and externally rotates the arm. It also stabilizes the humerus firmly in the shoulder 'socket'

Signs & Symptoms:

- The deep, aching pain 'caps' the shoulder and may extend down the outside of the arm. It may include the area of the arm where 'tennis elbow' is experienced.
- Pain increases with movement
- At rest, pain is dull ache
- Clicking or 'snapping' may be experienced during movement of the shoulder
- Restricted shoulder motion during sports such as tennis
- When attempting to raise arm out to side, it shortens the muscle, increasing pain

Causes:

- When heavy objects are carried, i.e., a suitcase, with the arm hanging down, or that object is lifted above shoulder height with the arm outstretched
- Walking a dog on a leash
- Weakness or lengthening of the lower trapezius for prolonged periods alters the position of the shoulder joint, requiring constant activation of this muscle
- Reaching up for objects above the shoulder
- Pain may increase when sleeping on either side at night
- Reaching to comb hair, brush teeth or shave
- Arm swing while walking may aggravate symptoms once TrP has become active

Refer to Index, Legend, Figures, Glossary & Abbreviations

Management Tips:

- Use a pressure tool on the TrPs that reproduce your symptoms
- TrPs may be active when joint is prone to subluxation, i.e., stroke patient
- Stretch by placing your arm behind your back and pulling the shoulder and elbow down as you reach to move your hand as far as possible across your back

Preventing Recurrence:

- Avoid carrying heavy objects with arm down at side
- Avoid sustained work overhead or at arms length in front
- Avoid repetitive, forceful actions, i.e., throwing a ball
- Use a warm up program before repetitive activity in sports, i.e., tennis, golf

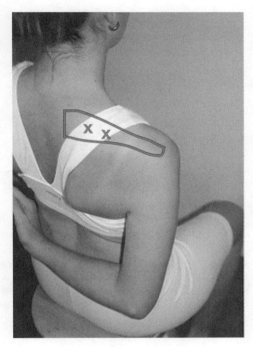

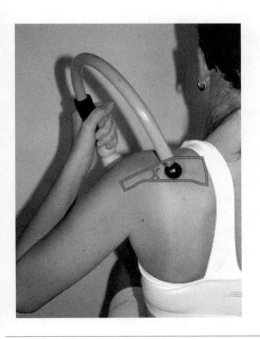

Check these TrPs:

Infraspinatus
Lower trapezius
Deltoid
Upper trapezius

Remember the rules for stretching and applying pressure

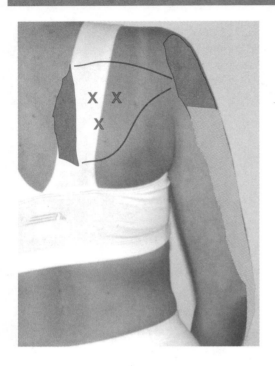

Related Dx's:

- Bicipital tendonitis
- Subdeltoid bursitis
- Frozen shoulder
- Cervical disc disease
- Arthritis in shoulder joint
- Overuse/Repetitive Strain Injury

The Muscle:

The <u>infraspinatus</u> and <u>teres minor</u> are responsible for external rotation of the shoulder and act as a stabilizer during other shoulder movements.

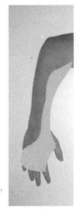
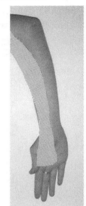

Signs & Symptoms:

- Deep, aching pain in the front of the shoulder is most common, as if the "bone were throbbing"
- Pain may also occur along the edge of the shoulder blade near the spine
- Increased perception of fatigue
- Increased sweating
- Changes in skin temperature
- Weakness in grip
- Reduced ROM in the shoulder
- Clicking or "catching" in shoulder with motion

Causes

- <u>Acute:</u> Grabbing backward to regain balance to stop a fall
- Excessive or sudden use of ski poles
- <u>Chronic:</u> Reaching backward and up while in bed
- Working for long periods in a static position when the shoulder blade is not stabilized
- Teres minor overworks when infraspinatus has been overloaded (fatigued)
- Reaching over head as in combing hair
- Putting involved arm in coat after your other arm is in the sleeve
- Sleeping on involved side

Refer to Index, Legend, Figures, Glossary & Abbreviations

Management Tips:

- Lay on the floor and use tennis balls to apply pressure to the TrP; gradually increase pressure by adding body weight
- When doing the stretch as shown, put the opposite hand on the elbow and assist the stretch by gently pulling the elbow toward the opposite shoulder
- Postural habit of keeping arm internally rotated will enlongate these muscles

Preventing Recurrence:

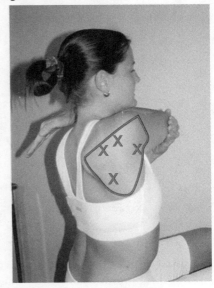

- When sleeping on the uninvolved side, a pillow should be placed under the involved arm for support
- Avoid lifting weights overhead
- When doing static or repetitive work the shoulder blade should be kept in place with strengthening exercises and pinching the shoulder blades together as a break during the work day
- Develop endurance & strengthen stabilizers of scapula

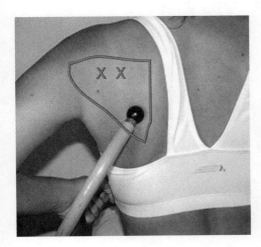

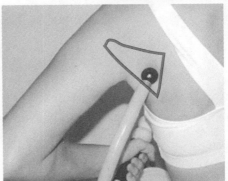

Check these TrPs:

Lower trapezius
Anterior deltoid
Rhomboid

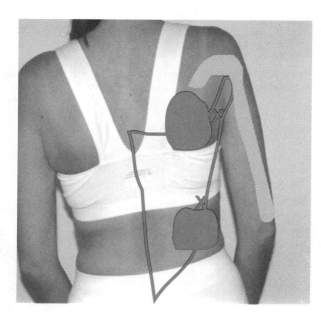

Related Dx's:

- Cervical disc disease
- Thoracic outlet syndrome
- Mid-thoracic backache

The Muscle:

The latissimus dorsi and teres major extends the arm at the shoulder, adduct and internally rotate the arm. Assist in scapular depression and retraction.

Signs & Symptoms:

- Pain at the lower corner the scapula and may radiate down back of arm into little and ring fingers
- Anterior shoulder pain
- Axillary pain posteriorly

Causes

- Reaching overhead with a weight in hand, overdoing; prolonged overhead work
- Swinging without adequate preparation, hanging from a swing or rope and gardening
- Reaching up or far out in front, as in handling a large bulk item
- Using a heavy tool at shoulder level
- Working for prolonged period with arms forward and elevated
- May develop from crutch-walking
- Overuse of arms to spare the low back

Refer to Index, Legend, Figures, Glossary & Abbreviations

Management Tips:

- Lying down on the floor using a ball on the TrP, adding body weight to increase pressure
- When tight the latissimus may limit full flexion and rotation of the low back

Preventing Recurrence:

- Use a stool to reduce upward and forward reach
- Place a pillow in the axilla between elbow and chest
- Support arms if forward position of arms must be maintained

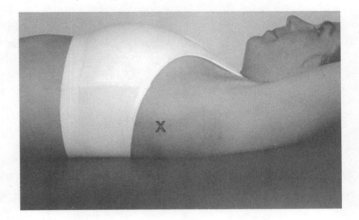

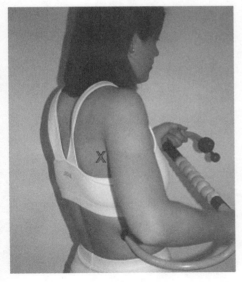

Check these
TrPs:

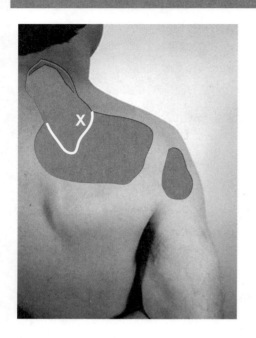

Related Dx's:

- Rhomboid & trapezius dysfunction
- Pinched nerve in neck
- Subscapular bursitis
- Carpal tunnel syndrome
- Tension myalgia of neck

The Muscle:

The <u>serratus posterior superior</u> assists with upper chest breathing

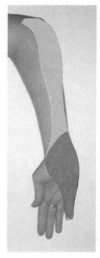

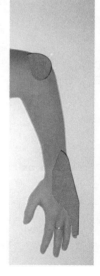

Signs & Symptoms:

- Deep scapular pain
- Intense pain over the back of the shoulder and upper arm
- Referred pain may extend to hand & little finger
- Tingling into little finger
- Deep, steady ache at rest
- Lifting objects with arm reaching up

Causes:

- Coughing from pneumonia, asthma or chronic emphysema
- Reaching to rear of desk top repetitively
- Posture that increases pressure of shoulder blade against ribs
- Sitting at desk too high with shoulders forward & rounded
- Typing with keyboard too high
- Chronic upper chest breathing; may be related to stress
- Scoliosis

Refer to Index, Legend, Figures, Glossary & Abbreviations

Management Tips:

- This muscle is a problem early in someone with CTD; work on the TrP early & often

Preventing Recurrence:

- Avoid overloading during breathing
- Postural support in lumbar region when sitting to maintain lumbar & thoracic curves
- Proper posture to correct forward head & rounded shoulders
- Take a break from tasks requiring static posture when sitting and using hands
- Eliminate upper chest breathing habits; learn diaphragmatic breathing

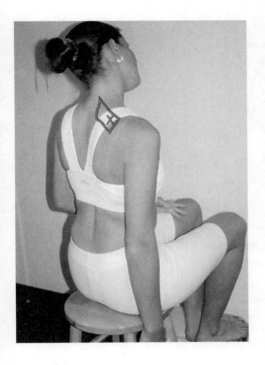
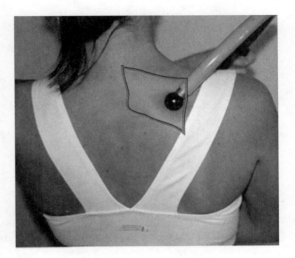

Check these TrPs:

Scalenes
Rhomboid
Infraspinatus
Lower trapezius
Upper trapezius
Levator scapula

Remember the rules for stretching and applying pressure

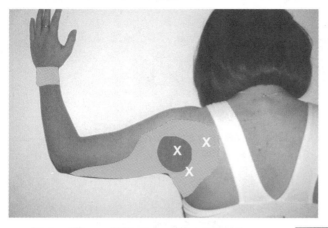

Related Dx's:

- Cervical disc disease
- Cervical spondylosis
- Frozen shoulder
- Autonomic dysfunction

The Muscle:

The subscapularis adducts and internally rotates the arm

Note: These TrPs are underneath the shoulder blade and cannot be reached by the patient.

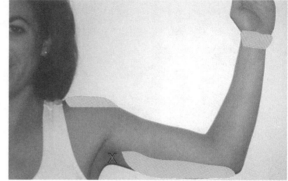

Signs & Symptoms:

- Pain occurs both at rest and with motion
- Pain is primarily felt behind the shoulder joint
- A strap-like referred pain area may be present around the wrist
- Limited motion in abduction and external rotation
- May not be able to reach across chest to other underarm

Causes:

- Acute: Reaching backward to catch yourself when falling
- Shoulder joint dislocation
- Fracture of proximal humerus
- Prolonged immobilization in a sling after surgery
- Chronic: Repetitive activity such as crawl stroke swimming when not in condition, or pitching action
- Forceful overhead lifting with strong adduction, as in picking up a child to place on someone's shoulders
- Attempts to lift a heavy object out to the side
- Immobilization due to pain, shoulder dysfunction

Refer to Index, Legend, Figures, Glossary & Abbreviations

Management Tips:

- This is one of the most difficult TrPs to reach. Lying on your back using a pressure tool may enable you to reach the TrPs without help
- Infraspinatus and Teres Minor TrPs may need to be released before releasing these TrPs
- Self management is limited due to position of muscle; may need to have TrP injections

Preventing Recurrence:

- Keep the elbow away from the body when sleeping on the painful side
- Support the arm on a pillow to keep it away from the chest when sleeping on the non-painful side
- Support the weight of the the arm when standing
- Move the arm frequently when sitting or driving
- Warm up prior to sports activities

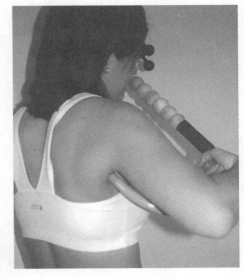

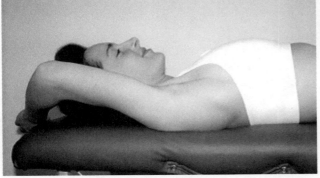

Check these TrPs:

Serratus anterior
Pectoralis major
Rhomboid
Infraspinatus
Teres minor

Remember the rules for stretching and applying pressure

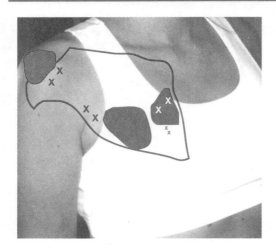

Related Dx's:

- Angina (chest pain)
- Pinched nerve in neck
- Subdeltoid bursitis

The Muscle:

The pectoralis major internally rotates the arm, protracts and horizontally adducts the arm

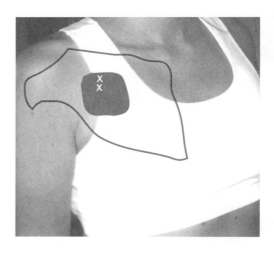

Signs & Symptoms:

- Pain over anterior shoulder, chest & breast
- Intermittent, intense chest pain
- Poor posture
- Limited shoulder abduction
- Irregular cardiac rhythm
- Breast pain

Causes:

- Long duration activities
- Sleep habits, position
- Attempts to abduct arm
- Poor positioning at desk or assembly work

Refer to Index, Legend, Figures, Glossary & Abbreviations

Management Tips:

- This stretch is done by grasping the hands behind the back and pulling your shoulders down and back, making the upper chest stick out (picture bottom left)

Preventing Recurrence:

- Avoid overloading in flexion, as in lifting heavy objects
- Avoid prolonged flexion position sitting
- Limit sustained scissor-type, repetitive grasping using pliers or cutting thick or stiff materials/objects
- Correct forward head, elevated shoulder postures
- Avoid sitting in chair without arm rests

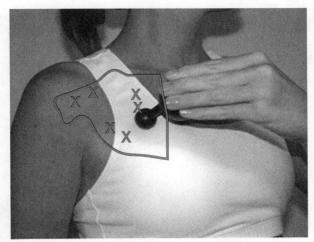

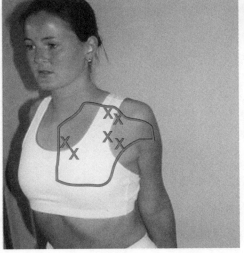

Check these TrPs:

Scalene
Anterior deltoid

Remember the rules for stretching and applying pressure

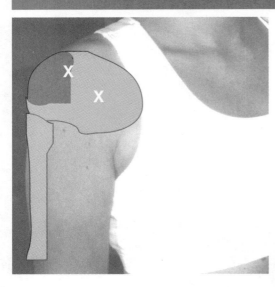

Related Dx's:

- Cardiac pain from lack of blood flow
- Costochondritis
- Pinched nerve in neck
- Subdeltoid bursitis

The Muscles:

The pectoralis minor & subclavius depress and protract the shoulder. Assists with deep upper chest breathing.

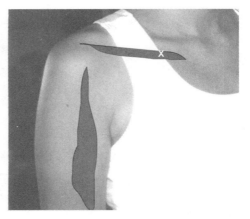

Signs & Symptoms:

- Pain over the front of the shoulder joint
- May extend over upper breast area or along inside of arm & ring &/or little fingers
- Difficulty reaching forward & up
- Cardiac arrhythmias
- May cause symptoms related to entrapment of nerves & blood vessels passing into arm & hand, with numbness & tingling in the arm, hand or fingers

Causes:

- Secondary involvement from other TrPs
- Overuse of crutches
- Poor posture with forward head
- Motor vehicle accident (whiplash)
- Compression from backpack slung over one arm
- Attempting to reach backward at shoulder level
- Attempting to pull shoulder blade back (retraction), stretching the pectoral muscles

Refer to Index, Legend, Figures, Glossary & Abbreviations

Management Tips:

- When doing the stretch below, the arm should be put on a wall or doorjam in the position of a hitchhiker's pose with the arm extended as far back as comfortable with the stretch felt just medial to the front of the shoulder joint. This position would not be acceptable if the front of the joint capsule is not stable.
- Stretching the pectoralis minor may temporarily increase entrapment symptoms

Preventing Recurrence:

- Correct postural problems at the worksite
- Reduce crutch walking
- Change gardening techniques to minimize forward, rounded shoulders, especially if pulling plants out of the ground
- Use of proper seating at home to reduce rounded shoulders

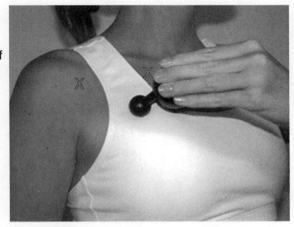

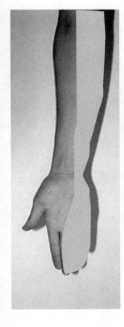

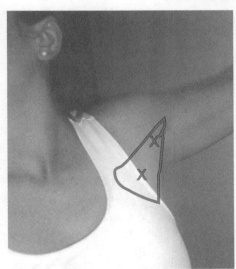

Check these TrPs:

Pectoralis major
Scalene
SCM

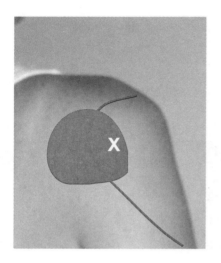

Related Dx's:

- Pinched nerve in neck
- Shoulder bursitis
- Bicipital tendonitis
- Rotator cuff injury

The Muscle:

The <u>deltoid</u> abducts the arm. Portions also assist with flexion and extension or horizontal abduction and adduction.

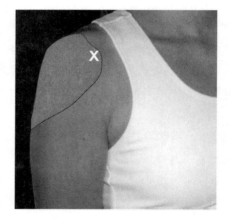

Signs & Symptoms:

- Pain is not referred from the TrPs, but stays in the area of the muscle and upper arm
- Pain is deep and aching
- Pain is greater with motion than at rest
- Decreased ROM of the shoulder
- Weakness in raising the arm out to the side

Causes:

- <u>Acute</u>: Impact trauma during sports
- Loss of balance and threatened fall
- <u>Chronic</u>: Typing at keyboard that is too high or too low
- Prolonged lifting or holding a tool at shoulder height
- Abduction of the arm with the arm rotated away from the body (external rotation)
- Carrying weighted object in arm

Refer to Index, Legend, Figures, Glossary & Abbreviations

Management Tips:

- Use hand held tool as shown, or lean against a ball on the TrP
- Use roller for deep stripping massage (see Ch. 17)
- <u>Anterior fibers</u>: To stretch, place your hand behind your back and then pull the elbow backwards (photo below right)
- <u>Posterior fibers:</u> To stretch, pull the elbow with the opposite hand, horizontally across the chest, feeling the pull on the posterior aspect of the shoulder joint

Preventing Recurrence:

- Appropriate ergonomic set up of work station
- Adequate stabilization of shoulder blade with appropriate alignment of shoulder joint
- Avoid repetitive activity of shoulder
- Use warm up exercises prior to use of shoulder

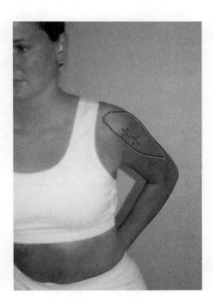

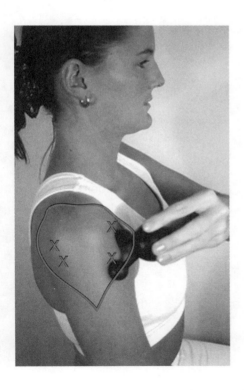

Check these TrPs:

Pectoralis major
Biceps
Infraspinatus
Long head of triceps

Remember the rules for stretching and applying pressure

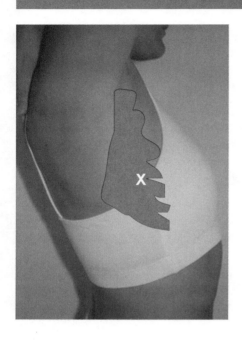

Related Dx's:

- Fractured rib
- Pinched nerve in neck
- Stitch in side when breathing

The Muscle:

The <u>serratus anterior</u> stabilizes the shoulder blade so the shoulder joint and arm are placed correctly for functional tasks. Helps keep shoulder blade against rib cage

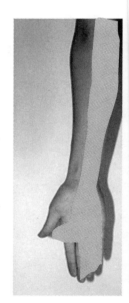

Signs & Symptoms:

- Pain under the arm on the lateral side of the chest
- Pain along the inner side of arm to ring & little finger
- Increased sensitivity over breast
- Pain with deep breathing
- Chest pain

Causes:

- Prolonged running or push-ups
- Lifting heavy weights overhead
- Coughing with respiratory problem (chest cold)
- Increased movement of rib cage, i.e., taking a deep breath
- Trying to pull shoulders back & shoulder blade closer to spine in correcting posture

Refer to Index, Legend, Figures, Glossary & Abbreviations

Management Tips:

- Press tennis ball against TrP and hold with arm until less sensitive
- To stretch, the arm is raised to 90 degrees, the elbow is bent, and the elbow is pushed backwards, so the shoulder blade "wings" (photo below left)

Preventing Recurrence:

- Correct breathing pattern
- Avoid lifting overhead
- Proper warm up program
- Strengthen muscles to keep shoulder blade positioned correctly along spine

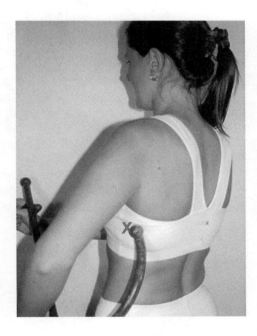

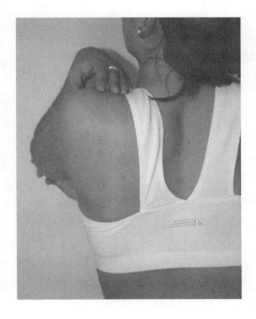

Check these TrPs:

Pectoralis major
Latissimus dorsi

Figure 16

Toronto, The Globe and Mail:

These quotes are from the article 'Pain therapy: An exercise in prevention'

Keyboard Grief. Coping with computer-caused injuries

Paul Taylor, Medical Reporter

"Ms. Headley believes that there is a logical progression in computer-related Repetitive Strain Injury (RSI). It starts with muscles in the back, followed by the neck and finally the arms and hands."

"What's happening is that the employee is put at a work station and basically uses just one group of muscles" Ms. Headley says. "Muscles were never meant to do just one thing for an entire day."

"Once the condition (RSI) has taken hold" Ms. Headley says, "you can't give every patient the same exercises. They have very different movement dysfunctions. And it takes some problem solving to figure out what exercise is going to create the desirable or necessary effect."

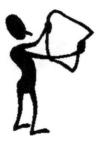

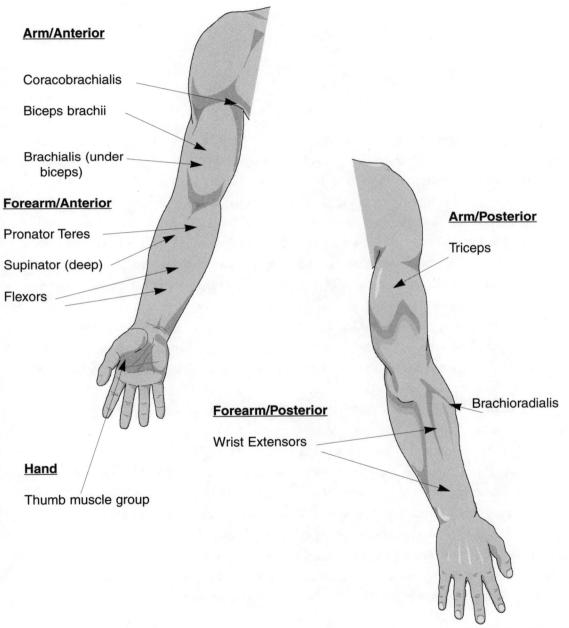

Arm/Anterior

Coracobrachialis

Biceps brachii

Brachialis (under
    biceps)

Forearm/Anterior

Pronator Teres

Supinator (deep)

Flexors

Arm/Posterior

Triceps

Forearm/Posterior

Wrist Extensors

Brachioradialis

Hand

Thumb muscle group

57

Chapter 6

Arm, Forearm & Hand Pain

Pain in the arm, forearm and hand can represent a wide variety of problems. Muscle pain may arise after immobilization for a fracture in any area of the arm. The pain of bursitis, tendonitis or capsulitis may also be accompanied by muscle pain. "Tennis elbow" is common, the problem found in the extensor tendons of the forearm at their attachment near the elbow.

Pain in the arm, forearm and hand may also arise from other areas of the body, especially the neck. In syndromes such as carpal tunnel (pressure on the nerve as it passes through the wrist), muscle and postural dysfunction in the neck may precede the development of actual carpal tunnel syndrome. In these cases, there may be proximal muscle pain and dysfunction in areas far distant from the area of pain that finally brings a patient in to see a physician. It is particularly important in such cases that the symptoms be traced back to their source, allowing intervention to be directed at the cause of the problem.

Pain in the upper extremity can be very limiting. It may be hard to open a jar, unlock and open a door, even sign checks when there is pain in the arm or the hand. The hand suddenly may feel very weak. Symptoms other than pain, such as tingling in the hand, or numbness, may frighten someone and be the primary reason why advice of a health care provider is sought. At the first sign of numbness in the hands the fear of "carpal tunnel syndrome" may be unleashed when often the symptoms can be relieved easily (if identified early) by release of TrPs in the neck muscles.

Pain Diagram

Using the concept of "being-aware", using the key on page 29, complete the body diagram on the previous page, filling in and labeling where your symptoms are being felt. This will help you to find the referral pattern of muscle pain that would lead you back to a TrP that might enable you to reduce the symptoms. Identifying where the symptoms are and learning how you might be able to control them is an important step in being a symptom manager.

The Checklist

The following list of questions serve as an initial incentive to think about what activities or positions change your symptoms. This, combined with other information, may be helpful in identifying the TrPs you should look for to try out your self management skills.

1]. Does the position of your head or shoulder alter the symptoms in your hand?

2]. What makes the symptoms increase in intensity?

3.] What have you done that has reduced the symptoms? How long does the effect last?

4.] When you move your neck, either to look over your shoulder or bring your ear down to your shoulder, does the neck move farther on the side opposite your symptoms during one movement or both?

5.] Do writing or other fine motor tasks increase your symptoms?

6.] When you stand and look in a mirror do your arms hang to the same level against the sides of your body? Is one side longer than the other?

7.] Do you look at your hand sometimes, wondering if you are still holding on to something?

8.] Do you sometimes find it hard to tell what you are holding in your hand?

9.] Have you dropped things like a cup of coffee from your hand?

Acute Trauma

When a person falls and lands on an outstretched arm there would be little doubt that a fracture was caused by the fall. While the fall or the fracture may not result in acute muscle pain, it is very likely that placing the wrist in a splint or cast for several weeks to allow the body to heal may result in muscle pain that increases when the cast is removed. Immobilization with the muscle maintained at a fixed length for a long time is bad for muscle. Part of this muscle pain is from using the hand in spite of the awkward cast or splint. The pain may also be due, in part, to the injury itself and the swelling that follows the fall. The pain that persists after the cast is removed is most likely due to compensatory patterns of movement and mis-use of muscle. For that reason, careful attention as to how you use the arm and hand, and from where the muscle pain arises can assist in reducing the residual pain that could become chronic.

Cumulative Symptoms

How often have we spent a weekend enjoying a sport or hobby such as tennis or fly fishing only to wake up the next morning with severe pain localized in the elbow, shoulder or low back? While we all might have experienced such a problem, it is also likely that we did not experience it after each and every tennis match or fishing trip. What makes this occasion different is not so much what you did on the trip, but what you had been doing for many months at work. You might at first not see that the assembly job you have, where you are asked to screw a part into a circuit board, for example, could contribute to your fly fishing pain. However, if the same movement pattern at the wrist is involved and you perform the repetition several thousand times a day, it may not matter that you have not been fishing in many months. It may matter only that you have done the same assembly job for five years. The same scenario may lead to pain on a Wednesday morning rather than a Sunday morning, leading you to the assumption that the only activity that causes you pain is your job.

What is most important to recognize is that many injuries occur over a long period of time although they may not be symptomatic, causing pain, until that final repetition that is the "straw that broke the camel's back". By recognizing the similarity between tasks performed at home and at work you may be able to avoid the development of the more chronic symptoms by looking at other ways to do some of the tasks, either at home or at work. One major difference is that at home you may instinctively stop doing the activity and "take a break", not allowing the pain to reach a very high level, while at work you do not have the option of taking a break. The symptoms, then, seem to develop only at work when, in fact, much of the repetitive task is being performed at home. By being a good detective you can alert yourself to these changes in your behavior, recognize their source, and develop good alternative plans of action.

Using this Section

Keep in mind that TrPs seldom occur in isolation and that you may have to look for TrPs in other areas as well. This generally means up in the neck and shoulder girdle for arm and hand pain. The original source of the pain may be quite a surprise to you. Use the "Check these TrPs" section to give you an idea of what other pages in the book may be helpful to you. You may need to be more creative and look beyond these TrPs.

Keep in mind also that the muscle pain in the neck causing the arm and hand symptoms may be due to a problem distant to the neck such as a leg length imbalance. When your interventions do not get the results you expect, you might have to consult a health care provider for a source of the problem far from where you have been experiencing it.

Figure 17

Denying pain is often not a healthy coping mechanism, and often leaves one feeling more out of control. Awareness of pain may lead to better control and use of self management skills.

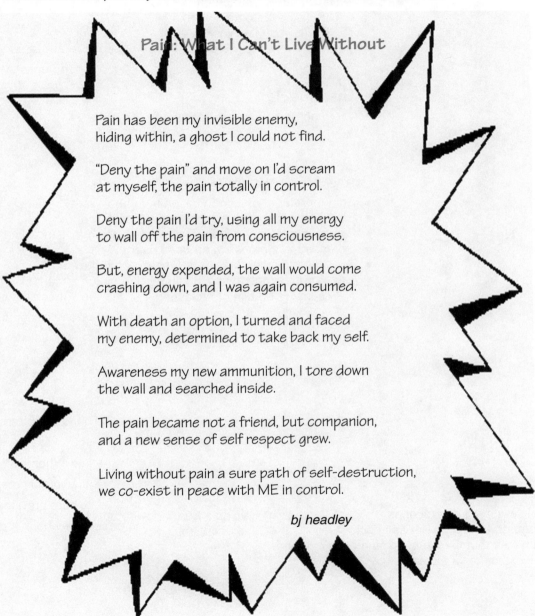

Pain: What I Can't Live Without

Pain has been my invisible enemy,
hiding within, a ghost I could not find.

"Deny the pain" and move on I'd scream
at myself, the pain totally in control.

Deny the pain I'd try, using all my energy
to wall off the pain from consciousness.

But, energy expended, the wall would come
crashing down, and I was again consumed.

With death an option, I turned and faced
my enemy, determined to take back my self.

Awareness my new ammunition, I tore down
the wall and searched inside.

The pain became not a friend, but companion,
and a new sense of self respect grew.

Living without pain a sure path of self-destruction,
we co-exist in peace with ME in control.

bj headley

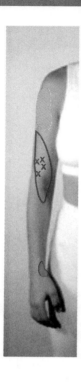

Related Dx's:

- Pinched nerve in neck
- Radial nerve entrapment
- Overuse syndrome
- Repetitive strain injury

The Muscle:

The <u>brachialis</u> flexes the elbow

Signs & Symptoms:

- Primary referral of pain to base of thumb
- Secondary pain over front of elbow & slightly above it
- Pain increases with elbow flexion & extension motion
- Increased tenderness in areas of pain
- Sensation of numbness or tingling over the base of thumb & web space to second finger due to entrapment of sensory branch of radial nerve

Causes:

- Heavy lifting, i.e., groceries
- Prolonged activity such as ironing
- Pain over thumb increased by motion of thumb
- Full extension of elbow
- Holding a heavy power tool
- Use of crutches

Refer to Index, Legend, Figures, Glossary & Abbreviations

Management Tips:

- Use roller tool or small pressure tool as in photo left below
- When stretching, turn the hand so the palm faces down and gently pull just above the elbow so the elbow is being extended fully (phote right below)

Preventing Recurrence:

- Limit weight lifted
- Keep palm turned up when lifting
- Use a pillow to limit bending of elbow during sleep
- Avoid prolonged elbow flexion

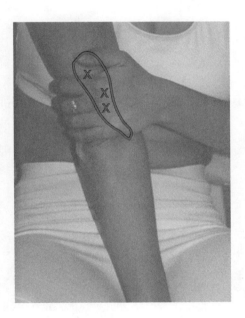

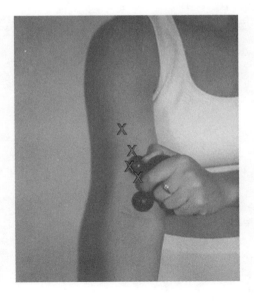

Check these TrPs:

Biceps
Supinator

Remember the rules for stretching and applying pressure

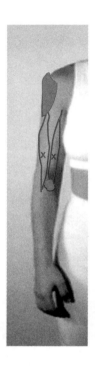

Related Dx's:

- Pinched nerve in neck
- Bicipital tendonitis
- Subdeltoid bursitis

The Muscle:

The biceps brachii & coracobrachialis perform shoulder flexion and the biceps flexes the elbow and turns the palm up

Signs & Symptoms:

- Pain reported in front of the shoulder and to a lesser extent in the back of the upper arm
- Pain considered superficial rather than deep
- Pain at rest
- Pain increases with abduction & elevation of arm

Causes:

- Acute: Catching a fall with the arm behind the body
- Chronic: Usually develops TrPs after loading of anterior deltoid, & triceps
- Biceps activity is high with continuous, rapid typing/data entry or turning a tool such as a screwdriver
- Trying to reach behind the back and across to the other arm
- Lfiting heavy objects with hand facing up

Refer to Index, Legend, Figures, Glossary & Abbreviations

Management Tips:

- Use roller or small pressure device (as in photo below left)
- Stripping massage may be helpful (see Ch. 17)

Preventing Recurrence:

- Eliminate lifting heavy objects with arms outstretched in front
- Lift & carry items with palm turned down
- Sleep with elbow protected from full flexion
- Good warm up program before repetitive/strenuous activity
- If using keyboard, keep elbow below the shoulder, at 90 degrees elbow flexion, and adjust keyboard location

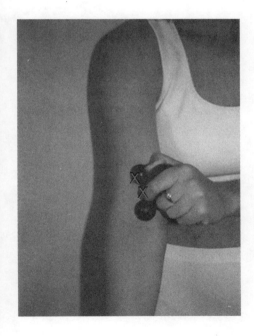

Check these TrPs:
Deltoid
Triceps

Remember the rules for stretching and applying pressure

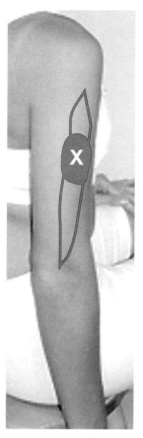

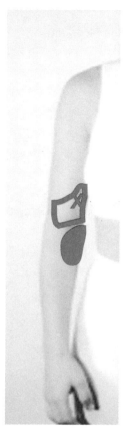

Related Dx's:

- Tennis elbow
- Arthritis in elbow
- Radial nerve compression at elbow
- Thoracic outlet syndrome
- Medial epicondylitis

The Muscle:

The <u>triceps brachii</u> extends the elbow & long head helps extend the arm

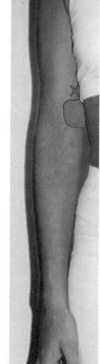

Signs & Symptoms:

- Refers hard-to-localize pain over the back of the hand, forearm & shoulder
- Pain referred over elbow with radiation to 4-5th fingers
- Lack of full elbow extension

Causes:

- Overuse of muscle when using crutches
- Sports such as tennis, golf
- Strong activity to extend elbow such as push-ups
- Activity that places arms in front of body for support for prolonged periods
  i.e., driving, needlepoint, quilting
- Trying to raise straightened arm up against ear may aggravate existing TrP

Refer to Index, Legend, Figures, Glossary & Abbreviations

Management Tips:

- Stripping massage would be helpful (see Ch. 17)
- Try placing roller on table underneath muscle and roll for deep massage

Preventing Recurrence:

- Increase use of armrest
- Keep elbow close to side, rather than reaching forward
- Correct arm rest height if length between shoulder & elbow is short
- Avoid overuse syndrome activities
- Maintain good scapular stabilization, with strengthening of rhomboids, trapezius

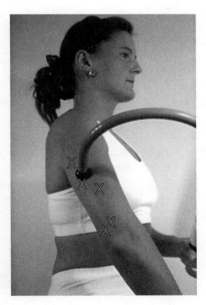

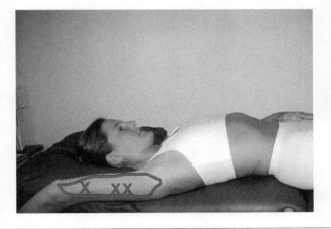

Check these TrPs:

Posterior deltoid
Teres minor
Infraspinatus

Remember the rules for stretching and applying pressure

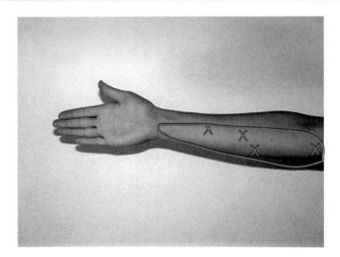

Related Dx's:

- Pinched nerve in neck
- Carpal tunnel syndrome
- Locking finger
- Tardy ulnar palsy

The Muscles:

The <u>flexors</u> flex the wrist and fingers. The <u>pronator</u> <u>teres</u> turns the hand face (palm) down

Signs & Symptoms:

- Referred pain to base of thumb, thumb or individual fingers
- Explosive pain that 'shoots' right out the end of the finger
- Difficulty using scissors
- Limitation of full finger flexor or extension
- Attempts to turn palm up with slight wrist extension & cupping of the hand may be limited
- Fine motor activity of fingers flexors
- Altered sensation in the 4th & 5th fingers

Causes:

- Prolonged static gripping of carpenter tools, ski poles, or steering wheel
- Fracture of wrist or elbow
- Performing manual therapy or massage with long static holds using fingers for pressure
- Excessive force while striking keyboard
- Racquet sports with inadequate scapular stabilization

Refer to Index, Legend, Figures, Glossary & Abbreviations

Management Tips:

- Use deep, stripping massage along full muscle length (see Ch. 17)
     - Start with superficial muscles and work deeper
- A hand held pressure tool can be used on each TrP (photo below, bottom)

Preventing Recurrence:

- Avoid or limit tasks that require prolonged forceful grasp
- Interrupt keyboard activity
- Maintain good position of the wrist when using tools or keyboard

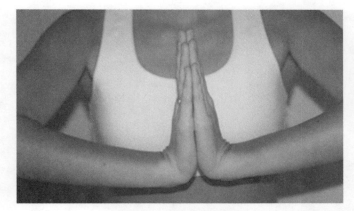

To stretch, place the palms together and slowly raise the elbows up. You will feel the stretch along the forearms in the flexors. One hand might be tighter than the other.

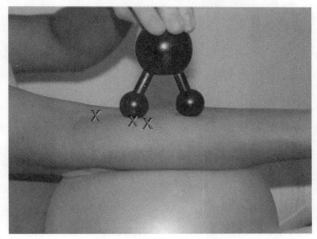

Check these TrPs:

Scalene
Upper trapezius
Pectoralis major
Wrist extensors

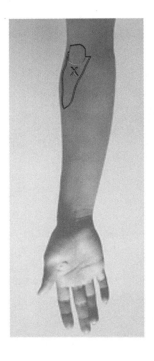

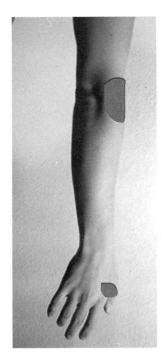

Related Dx's:

- Tennis elbow
- Briefcase elbow
- Dog-walker's elbow
- Radial nerve entrapment

The Muscle:

The <u>supinator</u> turns the palm up from pronated position

Signs & Symptoms:

- Twinges of pain over outer aspect of elbow or base of thumb on back of hand (web space)
- Pain with repeated flexion/extension of fingers secondary to entrapment
- Limited elbow extension
- Pain at rest

Causes:

- Carrying a heavy briefcase
- Sustained pronation (palm down position) of hand, as in typing or assembly
- Resisting pronation (turning palm down)
- Unscrewing tight jar lid
- Walking large dog pulling on leash
- Playing tennis
- Shaking hands
- Raking leaves

Refer to Index, Legend, Figures, Glossary & Abbreviations

Management Tips:

- Stretch the elbow toward maximum extension; the palm is facing down during the stretch (photo below right)
- Use small pressure tool (photo below left)
- Release superficial muscles first, working from skin rolling to deep stripping techniques (see Ch. 17)

Preventing Recurrence:

- Keep wrist as well as elbow slightly bent during tennis
- Carry briefcase in other hand or under arm
- Reduce repetitive wrist-rotation motions
- Carry packages with hands turned palm up
- Correct mechanics of tennis backhand and serve

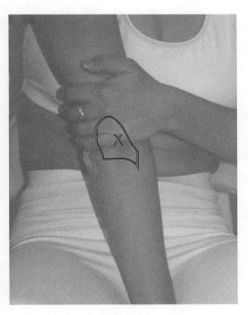

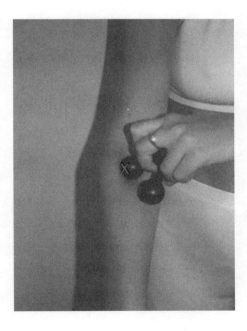

Check these TrPs:

Triceps
Wrist & finger extensors
Forearm flexors

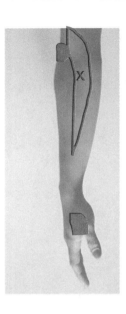
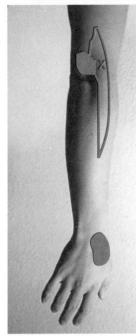

Related Dx's:

- Tennis elbow
- Writers cramp
- deQuervains
- Arthritis of wrist
- Deep radial nerve entrapment
- Arthritis of carpometacarpal joint of thumb

The Muscle:

The <u>brachioradialis</u> flexes the elobw, pronates and supinates the forearm<u> & wrist extensors</u> extend the wrist & fingers

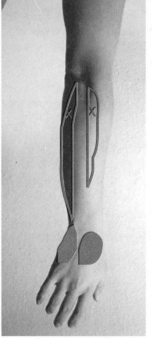

Signs & Symptoms:

- Referred to areas on the back of the hand and wrist
- Pain deep in upper arm
- Pain along outer aspect of elbow
- Numbness, pins & needles, painful vibration along the forearm to the thumb and index finger
- Pain with strong grip
- Dropping coffee, milk glass
- Objects slip from hand

Causes:

- Use of keyboard or handwriting at moderate to rapid rate
- Repetitive strong grasp with twisting
- Shaking hands
- Forceful grip with motion, i.e., using a screwdriver
- Loading or stretching muscles
- Typing
- Secondary to frozen shoulder or dislocation
- Entrapment may cause motor weakness or sensory numbness and tingling over dorsum of thumb and hand

Refer to Index, Legend, Figures, Glossary & Abbreviations

Management Tips:

- Pressure can be applied with hand held tool (photo below left)
- The brachioradialis is stretched by placing the hand down on a chair and gently straightening the elbow to its fullest range (photo below right)
- Stripping massage can be done, working from superficial to deep muscles (see Ch. 17)

Preventing Recurrence:

- Reduce or limit stressful twisting motion of the wrist
- Correct mechanics in tennis
- When movements are forceful, do not allow wrist to flex

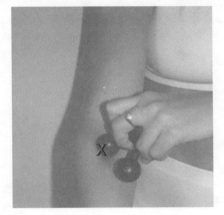

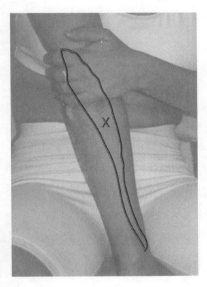

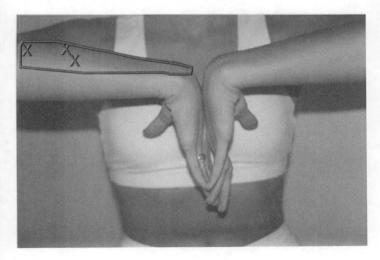

With the back of the hands and wrists together, the elbows are gently lowered (photo left)

Check these TrPs:

Supinator
Biceps
Triceps

Remember the rules for stretching and applying pressure

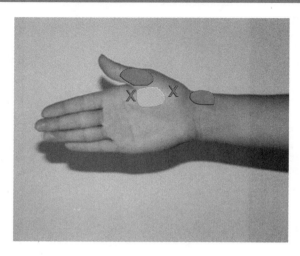

Related Dx's:

- "Trigger thumb"
- Pinched nerve in neck

The Muscle:

The <u>thumb</u> (thenar) muscles pull the thumb toward the index finge, away from the palmr & allow it to rotate to reach other fingers

Signs & Symptoms:

- Pain along outer and/or palmar aspect of thumb
- Complain that thumb is 'clumsy'
- Can hardly hold a pen
- Difficulty with fine motor tasks, i.e., buttoning clothing, painting, drawing

Causes:

- Use of tools that require holding muscle tension for prolonged periods when finely controlled activity is demanded, such as pliers, knitting
- Residual TrPs after bone fracture
- Weeding in garden
- Performing manual therapy or massage
- Trying to write long hand, esp. with ball point pen

Refer to Index, Legend, Figures, Glossary & Abbreviations

Management Tips:

- The involved muscles about the thumb can often best be massaged using the opposite hand or using a small hand held tool (photo below left)
- The web space between the thumb and first finger can be grasped and the muscle massaged if "knots" can be felt

Preventing Recurrences:

- Avoid persistent weeding
- Use soft felt tip pens rather than ballpoint
- Reduce muscle tension in thumb & forearm when writing
- Limit static holding, i.e., knitting
- Limit use of repetitve pinch tools

When stretching the thumb muscles, avoid hyperextending the end joint of the thumb by grasping the thumb in the middle and holding that joint while the muscles at the base of the thumb are stretched (photo right - should be held in middle of thumb)

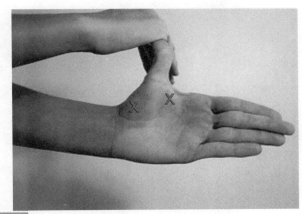

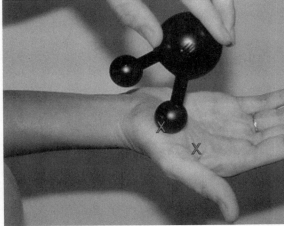

Check these TrPs:
Long flexors

Remember the rules for stretching and applying pressure

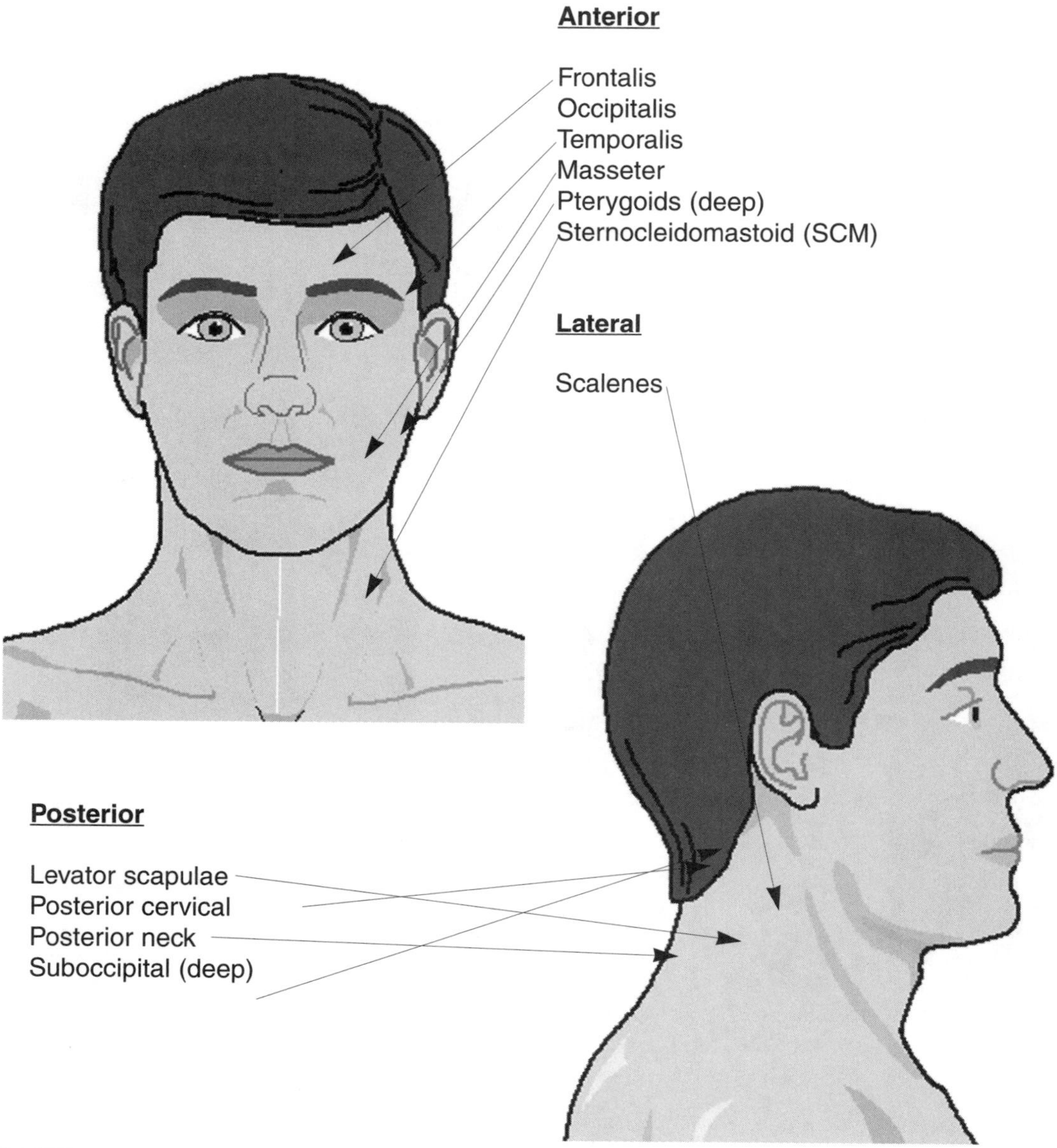

Anterior

Frontalis
Occipitalis
Temporalis
Masseter
Pterygoids (deep)
Sternocleidomastoid (SCM)

Lateral

Scalenes

Posterior

Levator scapulae
Posterior cervical
Posterior neck
Suboccipital (deep)

Chapter 7

Headaches, Neck & Jaw Pain

Many people think of headaches as being either due to muscle (the "tension" headache) or vascular (the "migraine" headache) pain generators. Many headaches classified as "tension headaches" are not associated with high levels of muscle activity, suggesting there are other factors involved as pain generators for these headaches. Most authorities would now agree that there may be vascular and muscular components to the majority of headaches. The various types of headaches would then exist along a continuum, representng a combination of factors that contribute to the headache symptoms. Many factors may contribute to the development of a headache including posture, stress, dietary and environmental factors. Identification of such factors is important in developing the appropriate self management techniques.

Pain Diagram

As with the other sections of this book, it may be helpful for you to identify where your pain is located before proceeding. You may then be able to look at the referred pain patterns and identify those that would apply to you. Using the diagrams on the previous page and the key for symptoms on page 29, complete the diagram before continuing.

The Checklist

Trying to answer the following questions may be helpful in identifying factors that give rise to your headaches, neck or jaw pain. While they may not all seem important at first, they may assist you with your problem-solving as you continue to read this section.

1]. Do your headaches almost always happen at the same time of day?

2.] Are your headaches related to any specific activity?

3.] Do your headaches come on after eating? Can you find any consistent pattern of foods eaten?

4.] Do your headaches occur when you are

most stressed out or tired? Stress can include positive as well as negative stress, as in the stress of putting together all the details of a wedding.

5.] Where do you first notice your discomfort? Is it in your neck, along your forehead, behind the base of your skull, or somewhere else? This can be a critical question for people with migraine headaches, as there may be a muscle "trigger" to the headache.

6.] Do your headaches come on after a long stretch of working, and when you have begun to relax?

Chronic Stress

Virtually everyone in an industrial society is subjected to chronic levels of stress. Despite all the advances in modern technology to make our lives easier and create leisure time, most people have less time for relaxation and vacation than they did 20 years ago. In addition, the advent of computers and their portability means that many business people no longer end their work day and go home; they simply bring their work home with them. Business people also work at the airport, on planes and every other minute they have.

Extra work time is now expected of salaried employees and often affects job longevity. Such work demands mean that for some people their work all too often is "never done" or they feel they are "never able to catch up." This presents a unique type of chronic stress that was not prominent in our culture decades ago. Previous generations experienced times built into the day when work was not possible, perhaps due to lack of daylight, or lack of help to complete the task.

Physical demands were much greater and much more variable in the past than they are now for most people, allowing variation to alter the imposed stress on the body. Fifty years ago people finished their chores and relaxed at night, perhaps doing small mending, cleaning or repair projects. The increase in serious sports training for children, for example, increases the stressful hours of planning and time management. The same can be said for dual income families and evening classes. Stressors were major threats to survival, not something they lived with every hour.

In our culture, there are fewer threats to survival, just a chronic lower level of stress that revolves around getting things done, financial challenges, and time management crunches. However, our body has one general reaction to stress. It is called the "fight or flight" response. It evolved millions of years ago, and reflects the simple choice our ancestors had - stay and fight the preditor or run. In order to accomplish either task, the body had to rapidly gear up for action. The sympathetic nervous system reaches a red alert during the flight or fight reaction, and the body is poised to act. Unfortunately for us, the same reaction occurs on a very frequent level in response to the small stresses we often encounter hourly. Instead of an emergency mechanism used occasionally, our body uses it all the time. Many of the responses of this fight or flight mechanism reside in the area of the head and neck, and constant activation of this stress response can lead to a stress headache. Clenching the jaw is also part of this state of readiness. Jaw clenching or grinding can become a chronic stress response with the onset of TMJ pain an eventual complication. While night splints may reduce the damage to the teeth, muscle dysfunction should also be addressed.

> Many of the responses of this fight or flight mechanism reside in the area of the head and neck, and constant activation of this stress response can lead to a stress headache.

abort the headache.

TrPs may also develop in response to the severe pain of the migraine headache. Muscles, tensed for hours during a migraine may not relax easily after the headache, leaving muscles vulnerable to the development of TrPs.

Vascular, Migraine Headaches

While the vascular component of the migraine cannot be treated with soft tissue techniques, in some individuals there appears to be a muscle that triggers the onset of the vascular component of the headache. In these cases, the muscle triggers should be addressed and treated, with keen awareness developed when the muscle dysfunction first appears, as early intervention at that point may

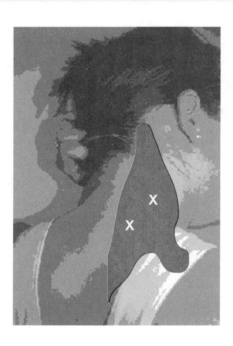

Related Dx's:

- Stiff neck
- Scapulo-costal syndrome
- Cervical sprain
- Cervical disc disease

The Muscle:

The <u>levator scapulae</u> helps to shrug the shoulder blade and rotate the shoulder joint down. Laterally flexes and rotates the head to the same side if the shoulder blade is fixed

Signs & Symptoms:

- Pain located at the top of the shoulder blade
- Generalized muscle tension headache
- Pain may radiate up near ear
- Neck flexion is limited at end range
- A 'stiff' neck with marked limitation in turning the head toward the side of the pain

Causes:

- <u>Acute</u>: Over-exercise such as crawl stroke when out of shape
- Vulnerable pre and post-respiratory infection
- <u>Chronic</u>: Prolonged activity with the shoulder in the raised or 'shoulder shrug' position
- Static work postures such as typing with the head turned to either side
- Holding the phone for long periods with the shoulder
- Sleeping with the muscle markedly shortened (as on a plane)
- Symptoms more likely if muscle is fatigued or exposed to cold drafts
- Walking with a cane that is too long, or sitting with arm rests too high or low
- Carrying a heavy purse or book bag on one shoulder
- Emotional tension, 'carrying the weight of the world' on the shoulders
- Holding on to anger or fear

Refer to Index, Legend, Figures, Glossary & Abbreviations

Management Tips:

- Direct pressure may be applied with a finger or a small hand tool (photo below right)
- The clavicle must be stabilized to achieve a localized stretch on this muscle. Grab the seat of the chair while doing this stretch while the opposite hand gently pulls the head down toward the opposite knee (photo below left)
- Return of ROM may be dramatic after proper TrP release

Preventing Recurrence:

- Face person or activity rather than turning the neck for sustained period
- Reduce sustained neck flexion by using a sloped stand while reading or writing
- Proper sitting posture with good trunk support and armrests to support neck and shoulder muscles
- Identify and correct possible vision or eyewear problem if forward head position while reading persists
- Carry items tucked under arm rather than slung over shoulder
- Use headset when on phone, or hold phone in hand

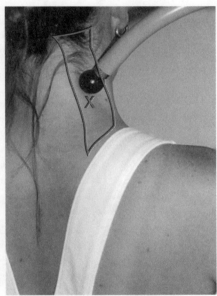

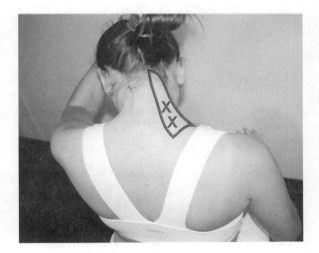

Check these TrPs:

Scalene
Posterior cervical
Upper trapezius
Serratus posterior superior

Remember the rules for stretching and applying pressure

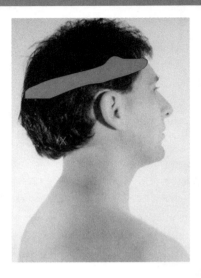

Related Dx's::

- Cervical pinched nerve
- Cervical strain
- Post-laminectomy pain syndrome of neck
- Tension headache
- Cervical arthritis

The Muscle:

The posterior cervical muscles extend and hold the head when it is slightly flexed

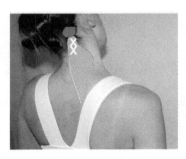

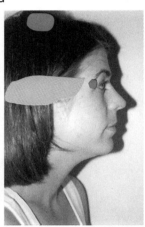

Signs & Symptoms:

- Pain at base of skull
- Pain resembling tight band around head
- Diffuse pain in skull from base of occiput forward to edge
- Marked limitation of head and neck flexion
- Tenderness on back of head & neck; may make pressure from pillow intolerable
- Numbness, tingling and burning over scalp on involved side
- Aching pain inside the skull
- Pain over neck and shoulder area
- Some restriction of rotation
- Pain at top of head
- Intense pain behind the eye

Causes:

- Acute: Whiplash
- Chronic: Poor postural habits
- Postural flexion from long periods while typing, sewing, reading
- Riding on stationary bicycle in a hunched over posture
- Cold drafts on back of neck
- Trauma, such as fall from horse
- Poorly fit and correction of glasses

Refer to Index, Legend, Figures, Glossary & Abbreviations

Management Tips:

- Use two tennis balls in a sock and place them under the base of the head while lying on your back
- Rollers work well, allowing you to do a slow, deep massage
- Use the double pointed end of the tool (photo below right)

Preventing Recurrence:

- Correct eyewear problems
- Adjust angle of glasses to avoid tilting head when using computer monitor
- Discard foam pillow
- Avoid reading in bed
- Postural correction of spinal curves
- Correct head position using computer monitor
- Avoid static position of head rotated to one side as in typing
- Reduce repetitive neck turning as when typing
- Correct set-up of work station, including monitor or assembly pieces

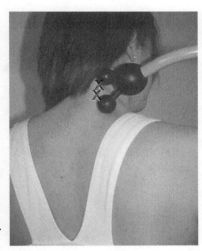

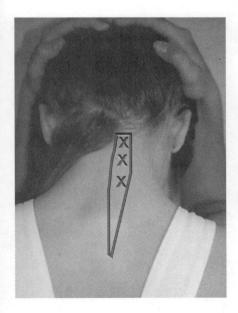

To stretch the upper heck, the chin should be brought down to the chest in the midline and to each side. The back of a chair may help stabilize the thoracic spine (photo left).

Check these TrPs:
Levator scapula
Upper trapezius
SCM

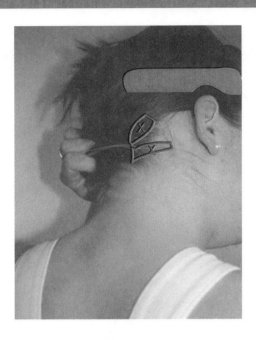

Related Dx's:

- Tension headache

The Muscles:

The suboccipital muscles, behind the base of the skull, span 1-2 cervical segments from the first two cervical vertebrae and the base of the skull. The alignment of the fibers is in three different directions.

Signs & Symptoms:

- Pain experienced deep inside skull, but not well localized
- Described as a headache "all over"
- May extend forward from base of skull over head to eye and forehead
- Will sleep on side to avoid pillow resting on base of skull
- Pain poorly defined at base of skull

Causes:

- Controlling rapid forward flexion of the neck
- Correction of eyewear needed causing difficulty focusing eyes on printed or small material
- Typing for prolonged periods with copy material laid flat on table
- Post traumatic headache

Refer to Index, Legend, Figures, Glossary & Abbreviations

Management Tips:

- Lie on floor on back and place two tennis balls in a sock under the base of the skull
    (These points are also considered acupuncture total body relaxation points)
- Flex the neck forward, turning the neck slightly and letting the chin drop toward the chest,
    stabilizing the shoulder by holding on to the chair seat with your hand (photo below
    right)
- Compliment these stretches with those of the posterior neck muscles

Preventing Recurrence:

- Revise computer station or other activity so head slightly tilted downward
- Place typing material on upright stand near monitor or attached to monitor arm
- Keep neck warm with loose neck clothing; may be necessary at night
- Computer monitor may need adjustable height and distance if contacts and bifocals are used
    at different times

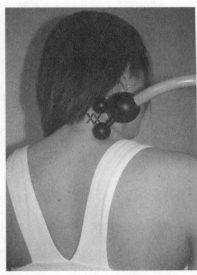

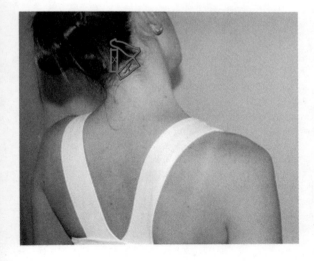

Check these TrPs:

SCM
Trapezius
Posterior cervical

Remember the rules for stretching and applying pressure

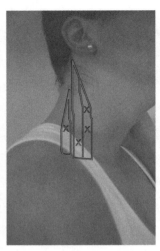

Related Dx's:

- Angina (left side)
- Subacromial bursitis
- Thoracic outlet syndrome
- Rotator cuff tendonitis
- Cervical disc disease
- Cervical strain
- Repetitive Strain Injury
- Carpal tunnel syndrome

The Muscle:

The scalene muscles assist in raising the upper chest during deep breathing. They stabilize the cervical spine. They assist in lateral neck flexion and rotation of the head (opposite side)

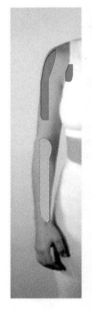

Signs & Symptoms:

- Pain over the anterior, lateral and posterior aspects of the shoulder and upper arm
- Pain over the upper aspects of the shoulder and shoulder blade near the spine
- Pain may also be referred over the back of the thumb
- Swelling may occur over the back of the hand (ring and little fingers)
- May report thumb as 'numb' when there is no change in response to cold or touch
- Hand swollen in morning
- Tension headache
- Disturbed sleep
- Limited neck ROM
- Numbness and tingling into the fingers may resemble carpal tunnel syndrome
- Phantom limb pain in upper extremity amputees
- Tightness in long extensors of fingers

Causes:

- Acute: Whiplash
- After neck surgery with front or side incision
- Handling reins while riding, or ropes while sailing
- Chronic: Prolonged forward head posture with rounded shoulders and poor scapular stabilization
- This may occur with aging and sedentary lifestyles, exacerbated by prolonged desk work, assembly, lack of regular exercise
- Prolonged accessory breathing as in asthma or upper chest breathing with low back pain
- A tilted shoulder-girdle due to short leg on one side, tight quadratus or short hemi-pelvis
- Forward leaning position due to short arms (resting on desk, etc)
- Entrapment of nerves and vessels in the neck when the scalene muscles are shortened by TrPs
- Postural correction involving the military stance

Refer to Index, Legend, Figures, Glossary & Abbreviations

Management Tips:

- The collar bone (clavicle) must be stabilized to get a good stretch (below center)
- The stretch may be done lying down, pulling the head with slight rotation of the head as well as lateral flexion (sidebending), i.e., looking over the opposite shoulder and up
- The stretch should be felt in the neck with minimal change in sensation into the arm

Preventing Recurrence:

- Raising the head of the bed (3-3.5") by placing blocks under the legs of the bed rather than trying to use more pillows
- Using headset or speaker phone rather than bracing phone by raising shoulder
- Rests to elevate elbows on desk
- Correction of postural asymmetry
- Correct eyeglasses
- Avoid forward head postures
- Reading without turning head
- Avoid pulling or carrying awkward packages
- Correct abnormal breathing patterns
- Postural correction with good scapular stabilization and postural alignment
- Use of cervical air pillow on planes or if passenger in car for long distances

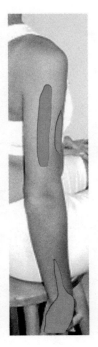

When applying pressure (photo right) be carefully located on the muscle, not underlying vessels

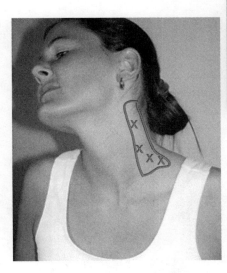

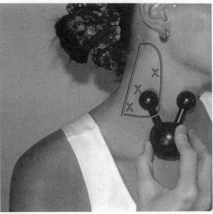

Check these TrPs:

Upper trapezius
Lower trapezius
SCM

Remember the rules for stretching and applying pressure

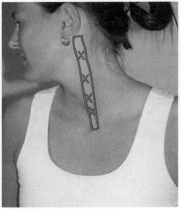

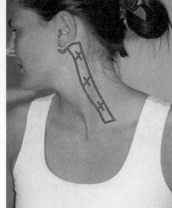

Related Dx's:

- Tension headache or migraine
- Atypical facial neuralgia
- Trigeminal neuralgia
- Sore throat
- Stiff neck
- Torticollis
- Meniere's disease
- TMD (temporal mandibular disease)

The Muscle:

The sternocleidomastoid (SCM) turns the face to the opposite side and lifts the chin toward ceiling; bends the face forward & down, assists with upper chest breathing

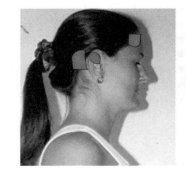

Signs & Symptoms:

- Pain around eye
- Pain just over eyes in forehead
- Ear ache
- Fainting (syncope)
- Paroxysmal dry cough
- Altered vision-blurring
- Altered sense of weight in the hand
- Dizziness related to posture and disturbed balance

- Pain in ear
- Pain in cheek and molar teeth
- Vertigo
- Upset stomach
- Weeping &/or redness of eye
- Cracking sound in ear
- Localized sweating

Causes:

- Acute: Neck extension for long periods, i.e., painting ceiling
- Whiplash/MVA
- Chronic: Scoliosis
- Chronic cough
- Compression by tight collar
- Sudden change of position of head

- Sports, i.e., wrestling
- Chronic postural compensation
- Hauling or pulling
- Leg length imbalance
- Rolling over in bed

Refer to Index, Legend, Figures, Glossary & Abbreviations

Management Tips:

- Anchor the clavicle and look over the opposite shoulder.
- Doing the stretch on the ball, clasp your hands together under your back to hold the clavicle down; let the hand drop back slowly by moving the ball and turn your head away from the side of the muscle you wish to stretch; do it slowly (photo below right)
- Do not do neck circles
- Go slow! Rapid stretching of this muscle or its TrPs may increase symptoms of headache, nausea, dizziness

Preventing Recurrence:

- Postural corrections
- Use headset or speakerphone
- Correct forward head posture
- Balance structural leg length
- Limit static neck rotation
- Limit overhead work

- Elevate head of bed from floor (3-3.5")
- Support of spinal curves when sitting

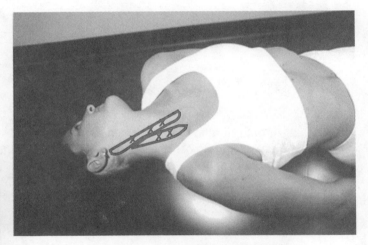

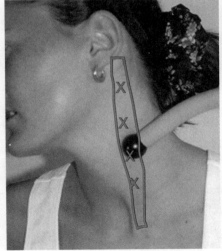

Be careful when you are applying pressure that you are on the belly of the muscle (photo left).

Check these TrPs:

Scalenes
Trapezius
Pectoral

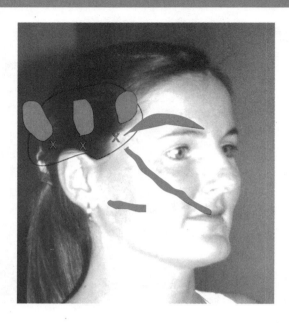

Related Dx's:

- TMJ disease
- Toothache

The Muscle:

The temporalis muscle assists in closing the jaws. Activity on one side pulls jaw toward that side

Signs & Symptoms:

- TrP toward front refers to top front tooth, other TrPs to top teeth on side of active TrP
- Headache pain is felt across the temple above and behind the eye
- Pain may be felt in some or all of the upper teeth
- Increased sensitivity to moderate temperature changes to any or all of upper teeth
- Toothache with pain from ordinary stimuli, i.e., biting heat or cold may be chief complaint
- May be slight decrease in jaw opening

Causes:

- High levels of muscle tension may cause the ischemia (lack of blood flow) that results in headache
- Bruxism
- Whiplash/ MVA
- Cervical traction
- Constant chewing
- Cold draft over muscle
- Clenching teeth
- Jaw immobilization
- Direct trauma, as in falling or being hit on head

Refer to Index, Legend, Figures, Glossary & Abbreviations

Management Tips:

- Hair pulling technique - See Chapter 17
- Severe sensitivity can be decreased by using a massager/vibrator very lightly over the area, slowly increasing pressure until other techniques can be tolerated
- Sensitivity common after whiplash or with chronic stress
- RubbingTrP with finger may be more effective than pressure tool

Preventing Recurrence:

- Malocclusion should be corrected
- Relax muscle by doing wide-open yawn
- Correct any postural asymmetries such as leg length differences
- Mouth splint
- Reduce stress factors

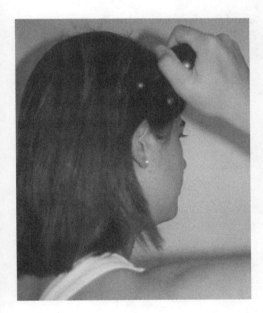

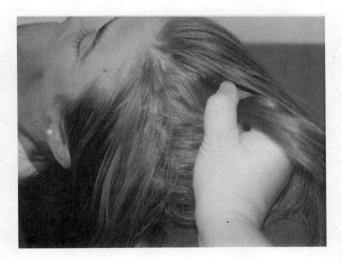

See hair pull technique in Ch. 17 to assist with release of this TrP

Check these TrPs:
SCM
Upper trapezius

Remember the rules for stretching and applying pressure

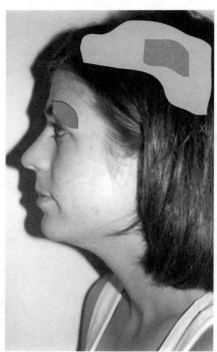

Related Dx's:
- Entrapment of greater occipital nerve
- Entrapment of supraorbital nerve

The Muscle:
The scalp muscles include the <u>frontalis</u> and the <u>occipitalis</u>. These muscles are most prominent in the front and back of the scalp. Together they can pull the scalp backwards, as in opening the eyes wide with fright. The frontalis can raise the eyebrow and wrinkle the forehead

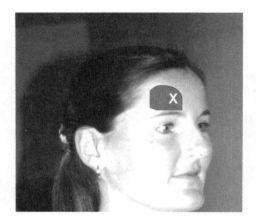

Signs & Symptoms:
- The pain from the frontalis spreads from above the eyebrow up and over the forehead
- Occipitalis pain is experienced diffusely over the back of the head and thru the cranium
- Occipitalis pain may be reported deep behind the orbit
- Unable to lay back of head on pillow due to occipitalis pain; prefer to sleep on side

Causes:
- Frontalis TrPs may develop from TrPs in the SCM
- Work overload, especially in tense people
- Maintaining worried or frown facial expression
- Occipitalis TrPs may develop from poor eyesight, poor visual correction or poorly-fitting glasses

Refer to Index, Legend, Figures, Glossary & Abbreviations

Management Tips:

- Use hair pulling technique as described in Chapter 17
- Use direct pressure on TrPs in the forehead (photo below left)
- Skin-rolling techniques on Frontalis muscle as described in Chapter 17

Preventing Recurrence:

- Avoid prolonged wrinkling of forehead or frowning
- Have eyewear checked
- Relaxation training for muscles' response to anxiety, general stress

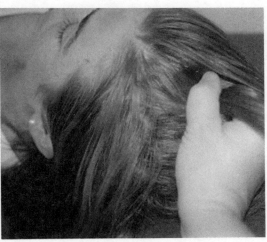

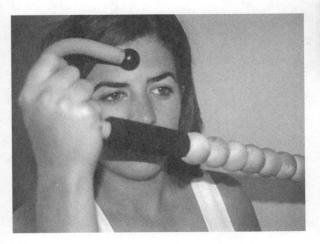

Check these TrPs:

Posterior neck
SCM

Remember the rules for stretching and applying pressure

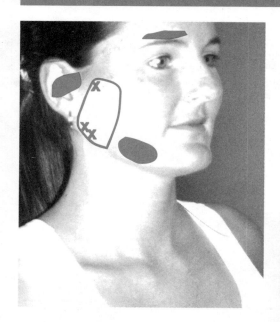

Related Dx's:

- TMJ problems
- Tinnitus
- Ear infection
- Tooth problems

The Muscle:

The masseter closes the jaws and is used in chewing or clenching the teeth

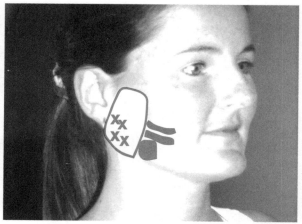

Signs & Symptoms:

- Pain may extend up over the eye
- Pain may refer to several teeth
- Incoordination of this muscle may cause irregular jaw movement
- Decreased opening of the jaw
- Pain deep in the ear
- Pain on the jaw and cheek
- Ringing in ear on involved side

Causes:

- Acute: Sudden, forceful biting as when chewing ice or cracking nuts
- Chin halter during use of cervical traction
- Chronic: Repetitive overwork as in bruxism
- Prolonged biting down on a pipe
- Extreme emotional stress
- Overstretching during dental procedure
- Chewing gum continuously
- Poor occlusion of teeth
- Secondary to TMJ disease

Refer to Index, Legend, Figures, Glossary & Abbreviations

Management Tips:

- TrPs can best be isolated by propping mouth open and using a finger inside mouth to press TrP from outside
- The jaw should be pulled forward manually as it is held open

Preventing Recurrence:

- Avoid exhaustive chewing
- Have bruxism treated
- May want to use bite block during dental work
- Hold mouth position as if saying "M"

- Decrease clenching habits
- Evaluate malocclusion

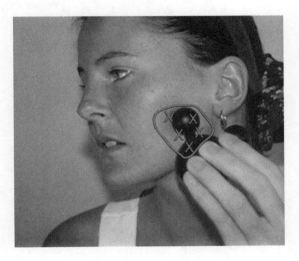

Check these TrPs:
SCM
Temporalis
Pterygoid
Trapezius

Remember the rules for stretching and applying pressure

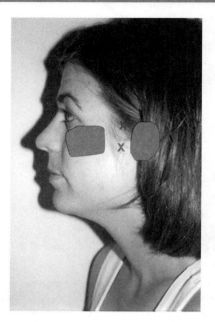

Related Dx's:

- TMJ dysfunction
- Sinusitis
- Malocculusion

The Muscle:

The medial pterygoid muscle assists in closing the mouth and shifting the jaw to one side. The inferior portion of the lateral pterygoid opens the jaw, protrudes the mandible and laterally deviates the jaw to one side. The superior portion assists in positioning the disc within the joint as the jaw closes. Both portions assist with closing movements when chewing with the molar teeth.

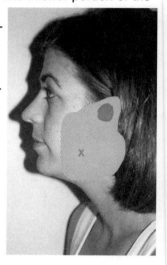

Signs & Symptoms:

- Pain in the TMJ
- Malocculusion
- Severe pain referred to maxilla
- Deviation of the lower jaw as it opens and closes
- Pain with tight clenching of teeth
- Ear complaints

- Clicking sounds & crepitus
- Pain may be poorly defined
- May decrease jaw opening

- Tingling in cheek

Causes:

- Bruxism
- Postural dysfunction
- Playing a wind instrument
- Excessive gum chewing
- Stress & anxiety

- Malocculusion
- Chronic infection
- Following motor vehicle accident
- TrPs in neck and shoulders

Refer to Index, Legend, Figures, Glossary & Abbreviations

Management Tips:

- Treatment of TrP can best be done by therapist or by physician with injection
- Stretch can be handled lying on your back on the floor, relaxing the jaw muscles, then grasping the point of the chin and with teeth slightly separated, rock the lower jaw so the jaw moves forward and backward

Preventing Recurrence:

- Correct occlusion
- Reduce bruxism
- Stop chewing gum
- Use of mouth splint
- Stress management
- Use bite block during dental work

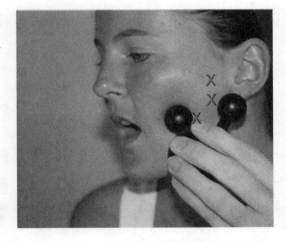

Check these TrPs:

SCM
Masseter
Neck Muscles

Remember the rules for stretching and applying pressure

Figure 18

Muscles & Postural Imbalances

These recordings are surface electromyography (sEMG), collecting information about which muscles are working during an activity. SEMG is discussed in Chapters 15 & 16.

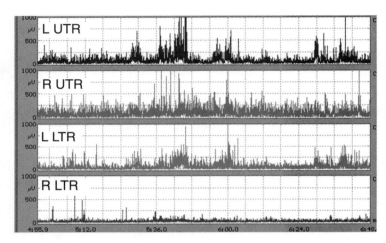

Carrying a backpack on only one shoulder (the left) results in postural and muscle activity which is asymmetrical. The shoulder on which the backpack is being carried is working harder, and so is one of the contralateral muscles. This same asymmetry is present when heavy purses or briefcases are thrown over one shoulder. The muscle activity is balanced and lower when the backpack is carried with both straps.

L UTR = Left Upper Trapezius
R UTR = Right Upper Trapezius
L LTR = Left Lower Trapezius
R LTR = Right Lower Trapezius

In this example, a patient post back fusion is walking with an SI dysfunction, creating a significant muscle imbalance and pain in the right buttock (L Glut).

L PS = Left L4-5 paraspinal
R PS = Right L4-5 paraspinal
L Glut =Left Gluteus Maximus
R Glut =Right Gluteus Maximus

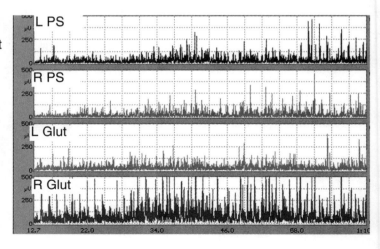

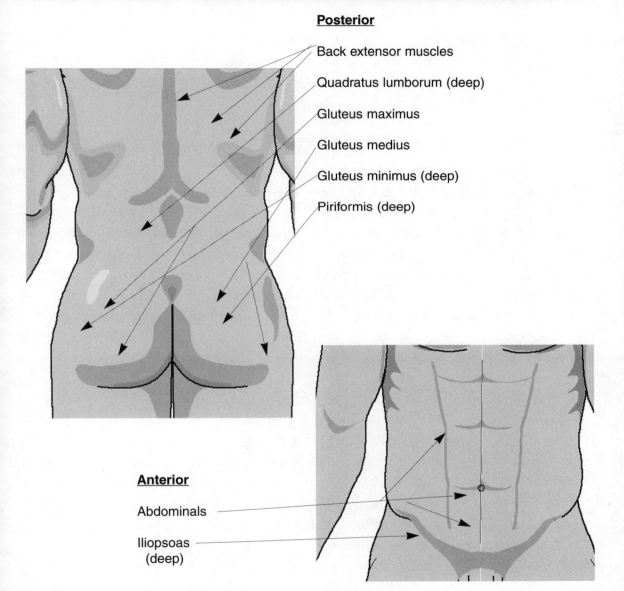

Posterior

Back extensor muscles

Quadratus lumborum (deep)

Gluteus maximus

Gluteus medius

Gluteus minimus (deep)

Piriformis (deep)

Anterior

Abdominals

Iliopsoas
(deep)

Chapter 8

Low Back Pain

People with chronic low back pain are given a wide variety of medical diagnoses. These diagnoses may include degenerative disc disease, herniated disc, mechanical low back pain, sciatica, facet syndrome, lumbar sprain/strain, failed low back and others. Many are simply descriptors of where the pain is located, but saying nothing of its cause, which is often TrPs. They may or may not have had surgery. If surgery has been done, a successful surgery may be well documented, but for the patient, loss of function and TrP pain may persist. Muscle dysfunction and pain are common denominators among many low back pain problems.

Muscle pain and dysfunction is often the result of TrPs and the movement patterns that develop after an injury. When can self management skills help with pain and how much relief might you experience? Some patients have learned that there is a lot they can do when they understand the impact TrPs have on muscle dysfunction. Given the proper tools, significant long term gains can be made in both function and symptom reduction. While self management skills may not mean that an individual will always be pain free, every minute, there is enormous empowerment in knowing what to do when, with the pain no longer controlling their lives. Like the other introductory chapters, a checklist may help you identify which TrPs to look at, and where you might initiate treatment.

Pain Diagram

Increasing your awareness about where and how your pain changes will help you use this manual. Filling in a pain diagram may help you decide which TrPs to examine. Use the diagrams on the previous page and the key for symptoms on page 29.

The Checklist

1.] What activities increase your pain more than others?

2.] Is sitting harder than standing? How does walking compare?

3.] Do you have trouble sleeping? What is your position of comfort?

4.] Do you stay in one position all night, or do you wake up and carefully roll over?

5.] Do you feel some times that one leg is shorter than the other, but it is not consistent?

6.] How well do you do on long trips driving or flying? What happens?

7.] Have you limited your activity to avoid certain activities? What leisure sports, activities or work related tasks have you removed from your life, avoiding the expected pain?

8.] Does your pain remain constant, or does it cycle with its ups and downs? Can you relate any position or activity to the changes in your symptoms?

Muscle pain is a common denominator for most individuals with chronic low back pain, regardless of medical diagnosis. As such, chronic low back pain can best be broken down by areas of pain and symptoms rather than medical diagnosis. Discussing them as such addresses the presenting symptoms and the characteristic patterns of posture dysfunction. It is these that generally contribute the most to limiting function. By addressing the movement disorder that accompanies chronic low back pain and the TrPs that may contribute to the problem, you have taken the first step in identifying the functional problem. Focus on solving the problem that limits function and causes muscle pain and postural dysfunction, rather than on curing the original diagnosis.

"Just Back Pain"

Limiting the pain to the low back, rather than including the legs, is not to suggest any lesser impact on function, or any limitation of suffering. The low back is central to movement. There is almost nothing that you can do without using your low back muscle,. including breathing.

If you have low back pain, think for a minute about how your diaphragmatic breathing may have changed as a result of your pain. Using the diaphragm means that as you inhale, the stomach will tend to protrude (stick out) slightly. As you exhale, the abdomen recedes. Good diaphragmic breathing limits the amount of upper chest breathing that is done, and is a more efficient method of breathing. Diaphragmatic breathing reduces the amount of adrenaline that is pumped into the body, as the upper chest breathing is part of the "flight or fight response". While upper chest breathing is not eliminated, the balance is what is important. Part of the diaphragm attaches on the last rib and this attachment provides its link to low back pain.

In an effort to splint and protect the low back to reduce movement of injured tissue, diaphragmatic breathing might be sacrificed. This further limits motion of the low back muscles. Limiting diaphragmatic breathing is a way to brace and protect the low back. The instinctive bracing of an injured area is important to reducing further injury. The problem lies in bracing this area of the body for a long time. If trying to breath with the diaphragm increases low back pain, the quadratus lumborum is the most likely culprit. This muscle also is often the culprit after an acute back strain. Stiffness develops as bracing the low back persists with functional and postural changes being inevitable. When the muscle is involved on only one side, that side of the body in effect shortens, and postural changes may develop that evolve into symptoms both near and remote from the initial muscle pain. These postural changes may also result in complex postural dysfunction (see Chapter 14).

> MPS might be THE MOST COMMON cause of low back pain.

Back pain usually includes buttock pain sooner or later. This may happen because of the changes in movement as one seeks to protect the back. Buttock pain also develops when secondary TrPs develop. This pain may extend into the central buttocks, or radiate to the hip and sacroiliac joint. Looking at the gluteal TrPs that may cause these pain referrals is a good place to start looking for answers.

Back and Leg Pain

The most common assumption about leg and back pain is that a disc has been herniated. Often, a subsequent assumption is that surgery is the only answer. And, in fact, such symptoms can be due to a disc and surgery may be necessary. There may be another answer, one which can be managed conservatively. It involves the most common low back pain culprit, the quadratus lumborum, but it also involves a muscle buried deep in the buttocks known as the piriformis. Through a quirk during intrauterine development, this muscle can put the 'squeeze' on the sciatic nerve. When the nerve passes through the muscle rather than under it. The nerve, once compressed, cannot tell you where the compression is located. Squeezing the nerve in the buttock will provide the same symptoms as if the nerve was being compressed by a disc in the low back. A good diagnostic workup may be necessary to first rule out disc pathology.

With irritation to the nerve, TrPs will inevitably develop along the leg. A gait pattern to compensate for the pain will usually increase the muscle pain along the leg and perhaps up to the trunk and the shoulders. Changes in how the muscles around the hip were used will perpetuate the muscle pain and cause it to 'spread.'

Other muscles will eventually become involved.

Sacroiliac (SI) Pain & Dysfunction

SI problems can often present as persistent pain in the low back and buttocks. The pain is often vague, hard to localize and characterized by deep aching. Sitting for any length of time is often impossible. SI pain may "come and go", making it difficult to be specific and track down the symptoms. Low back pain may not resolve until SI dysfunction is corrected.

Problems with the SI commonly follow lumbar fusions, often years later. They require evaluation by a skilled practitioner. Intermittent management is often necessary in order to keep the SI stable. Waiting weeks after symptoms start before seeking a skilled provider may delay stabilizing the SI and prolong low back pain unnecessarily. Self management skills can be learned with the help of a skilled therapist and are essential to long term stability of the joint.

Symptom "Spreading"

Many people with low back pain start with a very localized pain. In the acute stage, muscle pain may be limited to only one muscle. After time passes, and the initial muscle pain is not addressed, and the pain may appear to spread. Think about what might happen to your good posture if you had to walk around with one foot barefoot and the other foot with a high heeled shoe on. It does not take a rocket scientist to know that the back is not the only thing that will hurt if that pattern persists. Walking lopsided may cause symptoms to develop in the hip, the scapular area between the shoulder blades, the neck and may even trigger headaches. The sacroiliac joint may respond by moving slightly, and the weight bearing forces on other joints may be altered by the mal-alignment. Being a good detective is essential when the muscle pain has spread.

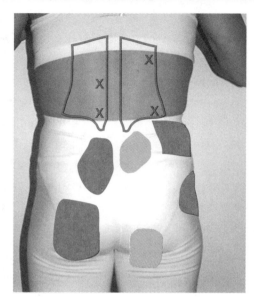

Related Dx's:

- Sciatica
- Trochanteric bursitis
- Pseudo-disc syndrome
- Failed low back syndrome
- Sacroiliac joint problems
- Arthritic spurs on spine
- Low back strain

The Muscle:

The <u>quadratus lumborum</u> has fibers that extend from the last rib to the iliac crest (posterior rim of pelvis) as well as attaching to the lumbar spine. The muscle acts to bend the trunk sideways, hike the hip and stabilize the lumbar spine

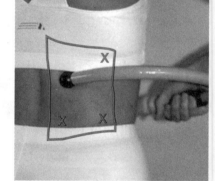

Signs & Symptoms:

- Pain deep, constant, aching at rest
- Pain radiating over buttock and into leg
- Sharp, knifelike when attempting movement as in rising from a chair
- Severe tenderness over hip (greater trochanter) may disrupt sleep
- Not able to stand up straight from chair without using hands

Causes:

- Sudden awkward movements
- Acute trauma, including motor vehicle
- Quick stooping with trunk twisted to one side
- Sustained forward trunk posture or repetitive bending
- Walking or jogging on uneven or slanted surface
- Sitting and having to lean to reach arm rests due to short arms
- Severity of pain may restrict all movement
- Increasing speed or trunk rotation while walking
- Often symptomatic after low back surgery, esp. fusions
- SI dysfunction
- Awkward lifting
- Coughing or sneezing
- Rolling over in bed
- Leg length differences

Management Tips:

- The stretch for this muscle is best done sitting on the floor (photo below right). If this position is not tolerated or you do not have the range of motion in your hips, sit in a chair that does not have armrests. Keep your buttocks on the seat of the chair
- With an acute flare-up, you might lie on your side with a small pillow under your lower ribs, gently stretching the muscle on the upper side of the body
- Pressure can be applied lying on the floor using a ball or tool, sitting in a chair and placing the ball behind your back, or standing using a tool (photo opposite page)
- This muscle, when short on one side, can make that leg functionally shorter than the other - keep it flexible

Preventing Recurrence:

- Determine if leg length imbalance is structural or functional & correct appropriately
- Learn how to compensate effectively for short upper arms or short pelvis on one side
- Develop proper body mechanics for lifting and avoid lifts beyond tolerance
- Treat trigger points early when it flares up with pressure and stretching
- Develop good sitting and standing habits with equal weight distributions
- Eliminate a sagging mattress; sleep with upper leg forward and on a pillow when on your side
- Use upright vacuum cleaner with two hands in front

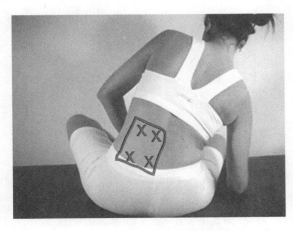

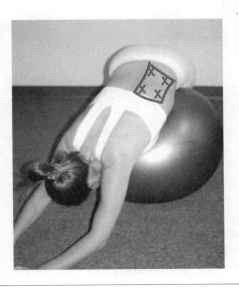

Check these TrPs:

Iliopsoas
Gluteal
Piriformis

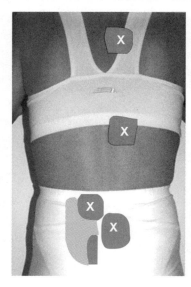

Related Dx"s:

- Angina
- Abdominal pain
- Hip disease
- Lumbago
- Radiculopathy with disc
- Coccygodynia
- Tumor
- Osteoarthritis

The Muscle: The long erector spinae muscles extend the spine, rotate the trunk and bend to the side

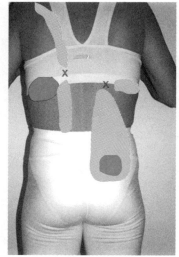
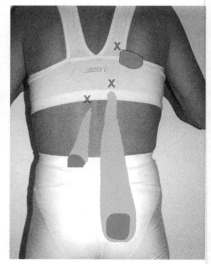

Signs & Symptoms:

- Buttock pain
- Unilateral hip pain
- Marked decrease in trunk rotation
- Unilateral bulging of muscle group in low back
- Unable to bend more than a few degrees
- Excessive to absent lumbar lordosis
- Difficulty getting up from chair
- SI pain
- Severe aching pain in "bones" of the spine

Causes:

- Acute: Sudden overload
- Chronic: Sustained muscle contraction
- Awkward bending and twisting of low back
- Whiplash/ MVA
- Leg length imbalances
- Prolonged immobility, i.e., seated in plane

Refer to Index, Legend, Figures, Glossary & Abbreviations

Management Tips

- The best defense against recurrent back pain is to keep these muscles strong & flexible
- Combine strengthening with dynamic stability

Preventing Recurrence:

- Correct structural dysfunction, i.e., small hemipelvis
- Use proper biomechanics, i.e., bending knees to lift
- Keep objects carried close to the body
- Provide proper lumbar support sitting
- Frequent changes of position to alter length/tension of paraspinal muscles
- Use Swiss ball or air cushion for sitting to activate muscles

- Correct leg length imbalances
- Firm sleeping surface

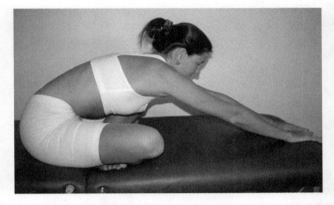

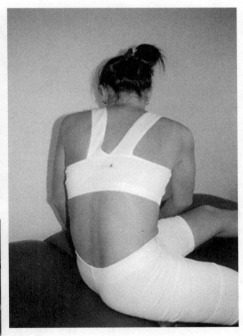

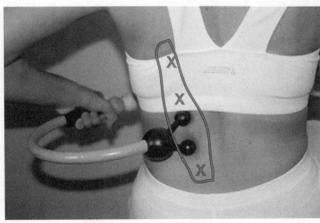

Check these TrPs:
Quadratus lumborum
Latissimus dorsi
Serratus Posterior
Superior & Inferior

Remember the rules for stretching and applying pressure

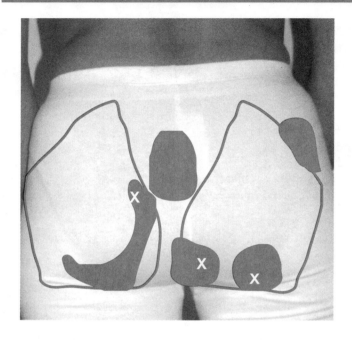

Related Dx's:

- SI joint dysfunction
- Trochanteric bursitis

The Muscle:

The <u>gluteus maximus</u> muscle is largely responsible for the bulk of the buttocks. It acts to control flexion when bending over or sitting down. It assists in hip extension and abduction, mostly when resistance is added. The muscle shows little activity with walking. It is active when the back is extended.

Signs & Symptoms:

- The pain may be localized over the SI joint
- Pain may be referred deep within the buttocks
- Pain may feel like a nail is pressing into the bone
- Walk with a limp (antalgic gait)
- Interrupts sleep

Causes:

- <u>Acute</u>: Overload stress during fall or near-fall
- <u>Chronic</u>: Prolonged uphill walking in forward bent position
- Leaning over from hips to lift (with knees straight)
- Sitting too long in one position
- Strong contraction in shortened position, i.e., swimming the crawl stroke
- Straight leg raise exercises prone or standing
- Sitting with wallet in back pocket
- Direct blow on one hip
- Morton's foot structure
- SI malalignment
- Donor site for bone graft

Refer to Index, Legend, Figures, Glossary & Abbreviations

Management Tips:

- Pressure tool may be used sitting, lying on floor, or standing and flexing hip (photo below right)
- May use ball while sitting or lying down
- The more sedentary your lifestyle, the more you will need a strengthening program for the entire gluteal muscle group
- Contract-relax technique works well when this muscle is painful and tight (see Ch. 17)

Preventing Recurrence:

- Postural changes when walking uphill or leaning forward to perform task
- Correct forward head position
- Stabilize any SI joint dysfunction
- Limit lifting that needs to be done with knees bent, as this increases the load on the gluteus maximus

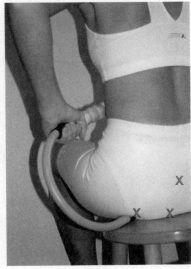

The stretch (below) is done lying on your back with the uninvolved leg straight. The involved side is crossed over and the pull and across (upper fibers) and across and up toward shoulder (lower fibers) without allowing the pelvis to rotate.

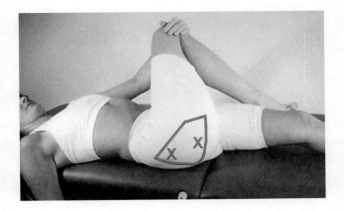

Check these TrPs:
Quadratus lumborus
Piriformis
Iliopsoas

Remember the rules for stretching and applying pressure

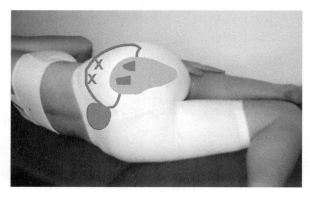

Related Dx's:

- SI joint dysfunction
- Lumbar facet joint pain
- Failed low back syndrome

The Muscle:

The <u>gluteus medius</u> muscle extends from the crest of the pelvis to the femur (thigh bone). It serves to stabilize the pelvis during the weight bearing phase of gait. It abducts the leg

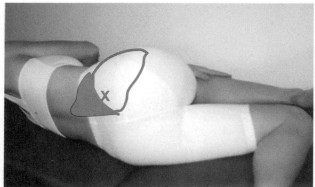

Signs & Symptoms:

- Pain may be felt over the SI joint and/or in the middle of the buttock
- May experience difficulty sleeping on the involved side
- Pain may be greater if one tries sitting in the slumped position
- Decrease in endurance during weight bearing activities

Causes:

- Leg length difference
- Sports, i.e., running, tennis, aerobics
- Long walk on the beach
- Injection of medication into the muscle
- Bone graft removal from the pelvis for surgery
- Lack of orthotics to control flat foot
- Carrying weight on one side of the body
- Morton's foot structure
- Sudden falls
- Wide gait pattern during pregnancy
- SI joint dysfunction
- Sitting with wallet in back pocket
- Often inhibited with low back pain

Refer to Index, Legend, Figures, Glossary & Abbreviations

Management Tips:

- Use pressure tool lying on floor, sitting, or standing (photo below right)
- Laying on the Swiss ball, the stretch shown for the gluteus minimus might also be helpful
- To stretch the more posterior fibers, the stretch postion should be modified so the leg is crossing over in front of the uninvolved leg, the knee bent and pulled up toward the opposite shoulder

Preventing Recurrence:

- Place pillow between knees and ankles when sleeping on side
- Avoid sitting too long. When driving, stop or use cruise control
- Do not cross legs when sitting
- Sit to slide on pants when dressing

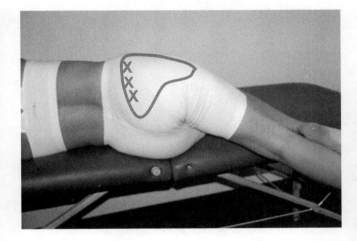

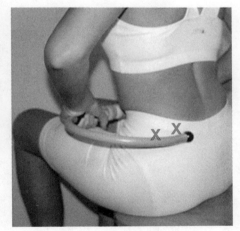

Stretching the anterior fibers of this muscle (above), lie on the uninvolved side and drop the involved leg off the side of the bed/table. The pull should be felt across the hip joint and pelvis on that side.

Check these TrPs:

Piriformis
Quadratus lumborum
Other gluteal muscles
TFL

Remember the rules for stretching and applying pressure

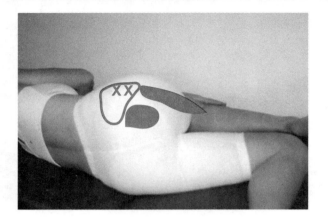

Related Dx's:

- Post lumbar laminectomy syndrome
- Sciatica
- Trochanteric bursitis
- SI joint dysfunction

The Muscle:

The <u>gluteus minimus</u> lies under the gluteus medius and assists in stabilizing the pelvis during gait

Signs & Symptoms:

- Pain in hip region may cause limp
- Pain may be constant and excruciating
- Seated patient may be unable to cross the affected leg over the opposite knee
- Numbness over pain referral pattern
- Refers tenderness over hip region

Causes:

- <u>Acute:</u> Falling
- SI joint dysfunction
- Injection of medication into the muscle
- Fast walking esp. on rough ground
- <u>Chronic:</u> Overuse in running and sports activities
- Driving a car for long periods
- Trying to sleep on involved side will cause person to awaken when they roll over
- Unstable balance standing, requiring additional stabilization
- Changes in orthotics

Refer to Index, Legend, Figures, Glossary & Abbreviations

Management Tips:

- The pressure tool can be used either lying down and slipping the tool under the butt, or standing (photo, below bottom)
- The stretch is done lying on the opposite side and dropping the upper leg behind and off a table; let gravity stretch the muscle, the leg slowly dropping down lower (photo below)

Preventing Recurrrence:

- Limit standing to short periods at one time
- Stand with wider base of support
- Sleep on uninvolved side & use pillow between knees and ankles
- Avoid or limit hiking or vigorous sports until TrPs under control

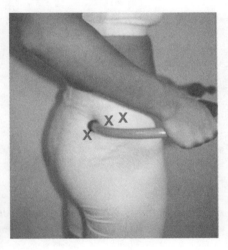

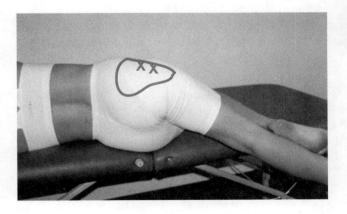

Check these TrPs:

Piriformis
Quadratus lumborus
Other gluteal muscles
Peroneus longus

Remember the rules for stretching and applying pressure

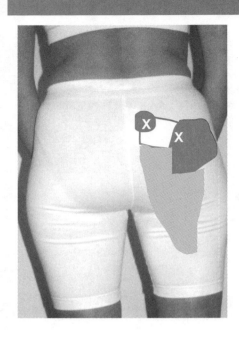

Related Dx's:

- Sciatica
- Lumbago
- Lumbar disc disease
- Post-laminectomy syndrome
- Coccygodynia
- Facet syndrome

The Muscle:

The piriformis is a thick and bulky muscle deep within the buttocks that externally rotates the hip when the hip is extended and internally rotates the hip when the hip is flexed

Signs & Symptoms:

- Pain is increased by sitting or standing
- SI joint dysfunction
- Mild foot drop
- Chronic pelvic infections
- Reduced sensation in low back, buttock, hip, back of thigh and leg
- Numbness in foot and loss of position sense requiring a broad-base gait and stance
- Pain when rising from sitting
- Gluteal atrophy due to entrapment
- Swelling in the painful limb

Causes:

- Doing a squat lift with a large object
- Acute: catching self during fall
- Twisting sideways while bending and lifting a heavy weight
- Forceful rotation with the body weight on one leg
- Tight quadratus lumborum on one side
- Chronic: Compensating for Morton's foot syndrome
- Prolonged sitting
- Sexual activity
- Following hip joint replacement
- Activation during car accident
- SI dysfunction
- Leg length imbalance
- Prolonged driving

Management Tips:

- A more gentle stretch can be done lying on side, with involved leg on top, flexing and dropping the leg in front of the other leg.
- Pressure tool may be used lying, sitting or standing (photo below right)
- Stretches may increase leg symptoms if sciatic nerve is entrapped until muscle releases

Preventing Recurrence:

- Correct leg length imbalances
- Limit driving time with foot on accelerator
- Avoid or limit strong rotation as occurs during tennis, soccer, volleyball or competitive running
- Correct gait deviation arising from Morton's foot syndrome
- Avoid sitting on one leg
- Reduce flat foot (pronation)

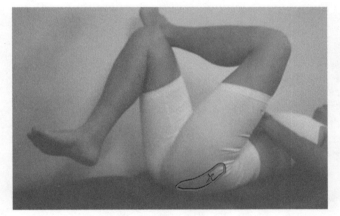

Supine stretch (left) is done by putting the foot of the involved side on the opposite knee and then using the uninvolved leg to flex the involved side until stretch is felt.

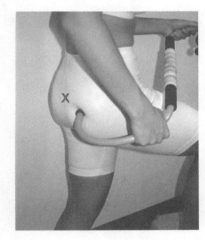

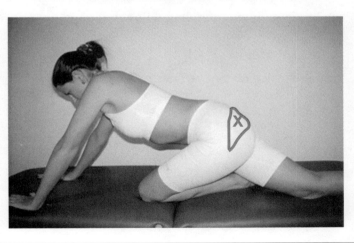

Check these TrPs:

Quadratus lumborum
Gluteal muscles

Remember the rules for stretching and applying pressure

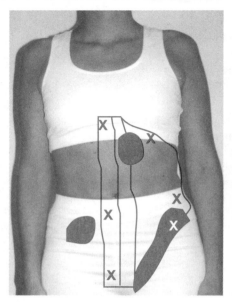

Related Dx's:

- Appendicitis
- Cholelithiasis
- Abdominal migraine
- Upper lumbar disc

The Muscles:
The muscles of the <u>abdomen</u> include the rectus abdominis and the internal and external abdominal obliques. These muscles flex the trunk, as in performing sit ups, rotate the spine, and increase intra-abdominal pressure. Fibers extend in three different directions from the ribs to the pelvis and to the midline abdominal sheath.

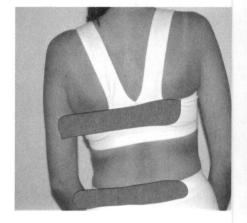

The referral patterns on the back are from the TrPs at the origin and insertion of the rectus abdominis

Signs & Symptoms:

- <u>Visceral:</u> Burning, Fullness, Bloating, Swelling, Gas Heartburn
- Groin pain
- Abdominal cramping
- Increased irritability of bladder muscles, producing urinary frequency, retention of urine
- Chronic diarrhea
- Pain referred to mid back
- Chest pain
- Pain to SI region

Causes:

- Acute or chronic overload
- Poor posture
- Leg length imbalance
- Total body fatigue
- Sustained twisted trunk position

Management Tips:

- You can massage the trigger points yourself by going to the areas near the origin and inser tion of the rectus abdominis; use a small, hand held tool (photos below left)
- Lying on your back over a Swiss ball would assist in stretching the entire muscl; slight changes in your position on the ball will change the portion of the muscle being stretched (photos right, top and bottom)

Preventing Recurrence:

- Proper performance of sit-ups
- Correction of postural dysfunction
- Correction of anterior pelvic tilt posture

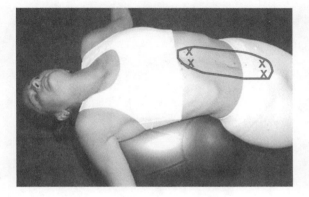

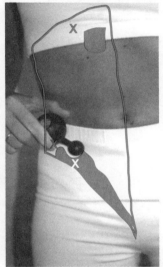

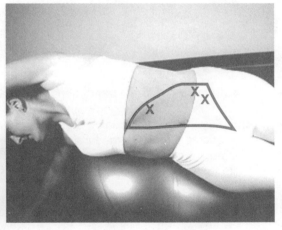

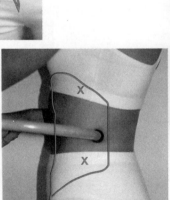

Check these TrPs:

Iliopsoas
Thoracic paraspinals

Remember the rules for stretching and applying pressure

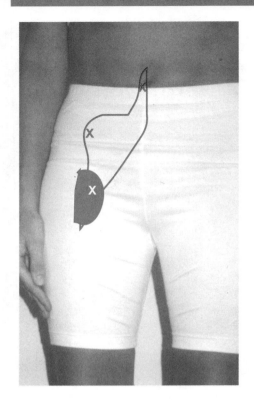

Related Dx's:

- Failed low back syndrome
- Appendicitis

The Muscle:

The iliopsoas extends from the lumbar spine and inner aspect of the pelvic crest to the hip (lesser trochanter). The muscle flexes the hip and arches the lumbar spine.

Signs & Symptoms:

- Pain extends in a narrow band along the lumbar spine
- Pain worse when standing upright
- Postural dysfunction, including stooped posture or forward tilt of the pelvis and increased lordosis (curve) of the lumbar spine
- Entrapment could result in decreased sensation in groin, upper thigh, or sexual organs
- Inability to stand up when getting out of bed in the morning

Causes:

- Leg length difference
- Acute: Activation with a fall
- Chronic: Sitting with knees higher than hips and leaning forward
- Pregnancy
- Prolonged sitting with hips fully flexed
- Post lumbar fusion with rigid gait pattern
- Walking long distances, increasing SI dysfunction
- Vigorous contraction during sit-ups

Refer to Index, Legend, Figures, Glossary & Abbreviations

Management Tips:

- Stretch must be felt in front of hip, not low back; back must be kept flat, in contact with table
- Supine stretch, pulling one hip up to chest and allowing other hip to lower over edge of bed, might be avoided if SI joint dysfunction is present (photo below right)
- Roll fingers inside lip of the pelvis at the location of the center TrP, gently massaging the sensitive TrP
- Kneeling stretch, keeping back flat with posterior tilt (photo, below left). This can also be done on a chair

Preventing Recurrence:

- Correction of leg length imbalances
- Correct muscle imbalances, e.g., shortening of hamstrings, abdominals, quadratus lumborum
- Restore normal movement of spinal segments in lower spine
- Re-balancing trunk's functional support, i.e., abdominal and low back muscles

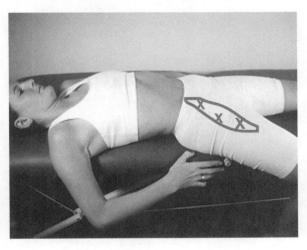

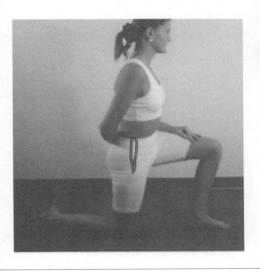

Check these TrPs:

Quadratus lumborus
Gluteal muscles
Adductors of hip
Tensor fascia latae
Hamstrings

Remember the rules for stretching and applying pressure

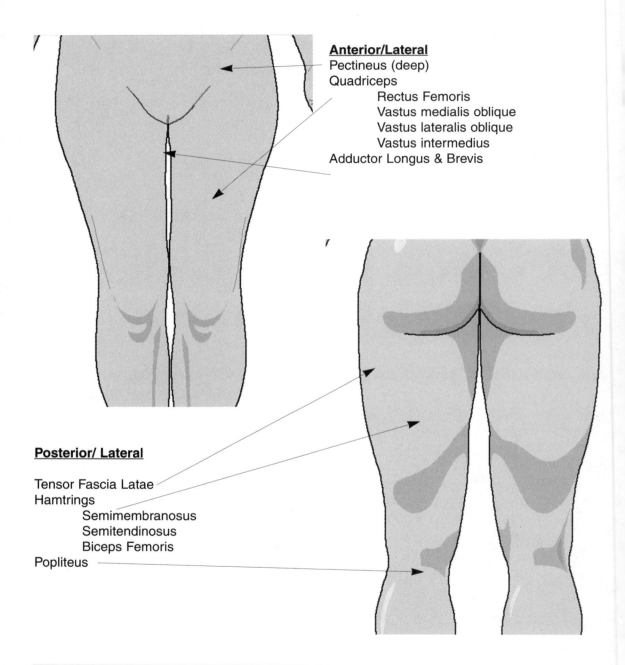

Anterior/Lateral
Pectineus (deep)
Quadriceps
       Rectus Femoris
       Vastus medialis oblique
       Vastus lateralis oblique
       Vastus intermedius
Adductor Longus & Brevis

Posterior/ Lateral

Tensor Fascia Latae
Hamtrings
       Semimembranosus
       Semitendinosus
       Biceps Femoris
Popliteus

Chapter 9

Thigh and Knee Pain

The dysfunction found in the thigh and knee can often be seen as the result of injury or compensation patterns that develop elsewhere. Certainly direct trauma to the knee can result in biomechanical changes and symptoms in the muscles that comprise the thigh. More often pain in the thigh reflects changes secondary to the low back and buttocks, foot problems or leg length inequality (either structural or functional). A checklist may prove helpful for you in sorting out how, when and where your pain presents itself.

Pain Diagram

Using the diagrams on the opposite page, and the key to symptoms on page 29, complete a picture of your symptoms. This will assist you in looking at the TrPs in this section.

The Checklist

These questions may help you determine which TrPs may be involved in your symptoms.

1.] Knee instability from old injuries may result in changes in the ability of the thigh muscles to work. Is the involved knee in any way "looser" than the other knee?

2.] Does your knee give way, buckle? If it does can you relate it to fatigue, long walks, stairs or any other activity or time of day?

3.] Back pain often results in thigh pain. Usually the pain presents itself along the back of the thigh but anterior groin pain can also be related to muscle imbalances in the back and pelvis.

4.] Have you ever been told you have a leg length imbalance or do you feel as if one leg is shorter than the other? You may notice it when you buy new pants, or have them hemmed. Leg length imbalances can be present all the time, or they can "come and go."

5.] Is the pain in your thigh constant or intermittent, does it throb, ache or is the pain sharp like a knife?

6.] Does the knee sometimes "lock" or get stuck on one position, making it difficult for you to bend or straighten your knee?

Thigh Bruises

Thigh bruises are often acquired during contact sports. Often these bruises are treated immediately after the incident. The individual resumes activity to finish the game and after several days of treating the bruise it is forgotten. It is not uncommon, however, for that bruise to alter muscle recruitment patterns of some or all of the quadriceps muscle, altering the biomechanics on the knee joint. This may lead to an increased susceptibility to knee injuries later.

Old Knee Injuries

Injuries to the knees also occur frequently during contact sports or sports where change of direction is rapid and frequent. After the injury heals it may be forgotten for years. A tear to the meniscus, for example, may heal without surgery. It may, however, alter the mechanics of the knee joint and a slowly increasing instability of the knee may occur over several decades. Suddenly a low back injury or painful hip may focus attention to the old knee injury, with careful evaluation of the altered mechanics necessary to understand subsequent injury development.

Even knees which are repaired surgically and identified as a totally successful surgery and rehabilitation may develop movement problems over time. This may mean that quadriceps function was restored but may not have been maintained. Involvement of movement dysfunction in the opposite (uninjured) knee may never have been addressed.

SI Dysfunction & Low Back Pain

Problems arising from the sacroiliac joint and the low back may result in pain referred to the knee from a variety of TrPs. The similarity of pain between the referred pattern of the gluteal muscles that mimics trochanteric bursitis and actual trochanteric bursitis may lead one to suspect that injection into the bursa is all that is necessary for symptom relief.

SI dysfunction often results in the development of several trigger points in the gluteal region that refer pain to the thigh. When SI dysfunction has not been recognized and treated for a long time, the dysfunction it creates alters the mechanical forces on the knee joint, perhaps increasing the susceptibility of this joint to injury. SI dysfunction radiates a vague, diffuse pain, often into the groin and back of the thighs that is very difficult to pinpoint. The pain is often aggravated by changes in position or sitting for long periods of time. In these cases, the thigh pain or eventual knee problems are secondary to dysfunction in the SI joint.

Low back pain often follows or precedes SI dysfunction and the low back is often the primary source of dysfunction when thigh pain is present. The signs and symptoms of the various problems can be sorted out by a health care professional skilled in the evaluation of low back, SI and knee problems.

cies and foot mechanics that may require orthotics may be necessary, and may resolve the thigh pain.

Leg Length Inequality

Leg length differences is a recurring topic in the book. The importance of length leg inequality cannot be overestimated. The difference in leg length may be present for a time, often decades, before problems begin to arise. This is discussed at greater length in the section on chronic postural stresses.

Leg length inequality may also result in damage to one knee. When one knee joint develops osteoarthritis much more severely than the opposite knee, mechanical forces or old injuries are usually involved. Leg length inequality may be structural (difference in actual length of bones) or functional (due to changes in mechanics, e.g., pronation of foot, SI dysfunction), and careful evaluation must be done before any lifts are placed in shoes.

Using this Section

As always, filling out a body diagram may help you focus on where the pain is located, and may help in looking at the referred pain patterns in this section. Single TrPs are seldom present when the pain has become chronic and other areas may need to be explored. A complete evaluation for both leg length discrepan-

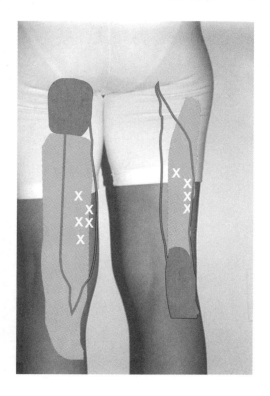

Related Dx's:

- Sciatica
- Osteoarthritis of knee
- Muscle tears
- Post-laminectomy pain syndrome

The Muscle:

The hamstring group of muscles act as hip extensors and knee flexors, and control the forward swing of the leg during walking

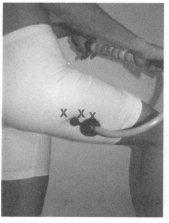

Signs & Symptoms:

- Pain may be concentrated at lower aspect of buttock, or behind knee
- Muscle inhibition may result in decreased hip stability
- Disturbs sleep
- Forward head posture
- Posterior pelvic tilt
- Tingling and numbness

Causes:

- Pressure on thigh from high edge of chair seat
- Prolonged bed rest with knees flexed
- Sprinting, kicking soccer ball and gymnastics
- Short statured people sitting in poorly fitting chairs
- Getting up from chair, esp. if one leg has been crossed over another
- Pain increased during exercise, walking downstairs, or with marked knee bending
- Overuse secondary to muscle dysfunction after low back surgery
- Small hemipelvis
- Lying on side
- Sitting and walking

Refer to Index, Legend, Figures, Glossary & Abbreviations

Management Tips:

- If very sensitive, use tennis ball to decrease sensitivity before using firm pressure or roller tool; soften the ball on the tool with foam, etc. (photo below)

Preventing Recurrence:

- Avoid repetitive crawl stroke when swimming or biking with seat too low
- Break up driving or sitting still for long periods of time
- Select chairs that match leg length or using angled foot rest

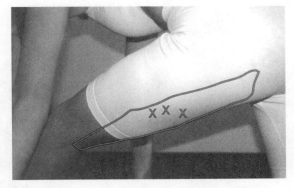

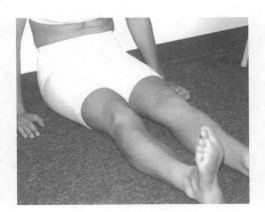

Stretch sitting on floor against wall (left), gradually straightening knees, keeping back flat against wall, or with leg out in front and reaching for the ankle (above).

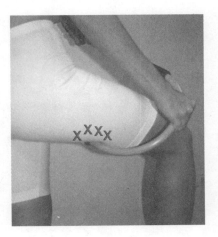

Check these TrPs:

Piriformis
Gluteal medius
Quadratus lumborus

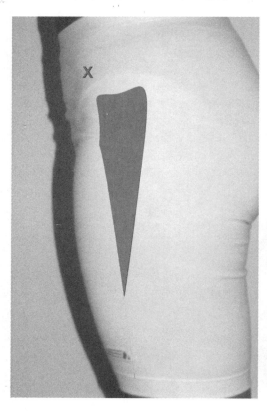

Related Dx's:

- Trochanteric bursitis
- Iliotibial band friction syndrome
- Arthritis of the SI

The Muscle:

The tensor fascia latae (TFL) acts to flex and abduct the hip and stabilize the pelvis during weight bearing

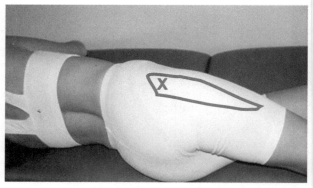

Signs & Symptoms:

- Pain prevents walking rapidly
- Pain referred to hip joint with tenderness over the greater trochanter
- Difficult to get leg fully straight after sitting

Causes:

- Acute: Sudden trauma such as landing on feet from a jump
- Chronic: Flat (pronated) foot
- Morton's foot structure
- Lying on the involved side
- Flat (pronated) feet, esp. in runners, may contribute to iliotibial band syndrome
- Difficulty leaning backward and hyperextending the hip due to increased pain
- Muscle imbalance with tight quadratus lumborum and weak gluteus medius
- Muscle compensation with TFL being used to flex hip without other prime movers

Refer to Index, Legend, Figures, Glossary & Abbreviations

Management Tips:

- Stripping massage using roller tool (phote below right and Ch. 17)
- Use pressure tool over multiple trigger points
- Roll gently onto tennis ball with tolerable weight gradually increased
- Densensitize with vibrator before using direct pressure
- When doing standing stretch of TFL and iliotibial band, reach for the outer aspect of the ankle on leg where muscle is being stretched (photo below left)

Preventing Recurrence:

- Avoid sitting cross-legged
- Avoid long sitting as in driving
- Do not run on sloped surfaces
- Keep hip extended during sleep
- Avoid walking or jogging up hills
- Gently stretch hip into external rotation each time you assume the standing position
- Alter seating surface so the front of seat slopes down compared to back of seat

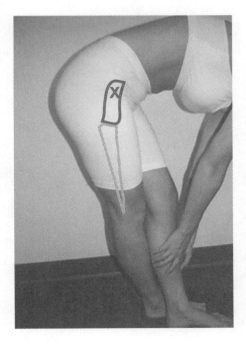

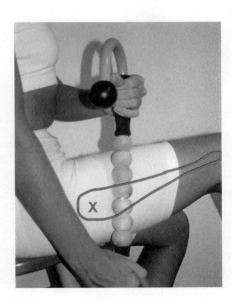

Check these TrPs:
Quadratus lumborum
Gluteal muscles
Iliopsoas

Remember the rules for stretching and applying pressure

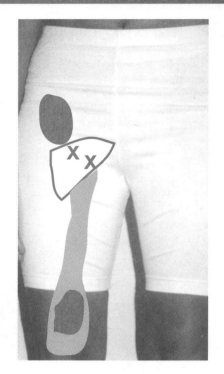

Related Dx's:

- Bilateral pain may simulate mid-lumbar spinal lesion.
- Pubic stress fracture
- Adductior insertion avulsion syndrome
- Osteoarthritis of hip

The Muscle:

The adductor longus, magnus and brevis adduct leg
Helps provide stability and lateral shift during the stance
phase of walking

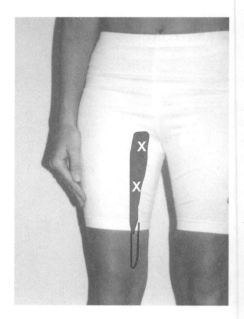

Signs & Symptoms:

- Groin pain is described as deep; often unable to localize pain
- May experience generalized internal pelvic pain, which may shoot up into pelvis and 'explode'
- Complaint of intrapelvic pain

Causes:

- Acute: Strenuous horseback riding
- Entrapment of genitofemoral nerve
- Chronic: In athletes, may co-exist with other problems
- Vigorous activity and twisting of the hip increases pain
- Weight bearing
- Aggravated by running up or down hill
- Sitting in fixed position while driving
- Sudden slips (on ice)
- Skiing or unaccustomed long bike trip

Refer to Index, Legend, Figures, Glossary & Abbreviations

Management Tips:

- Use of soft ball (tennis) before using pressure tool may help in sensitive areas
- Roller tool may help area to be less sensitive before working on TrPs (photo below left)
- Support knee during stretch to help relax muscle (photo below right)

Preventing Recurrence:

- Avoid leaving muscle in shortened position
- Limit the crossing of one leg over another when sitting
- Sitting in car for long time should be limited if position cannot be changed; get out of car frequently

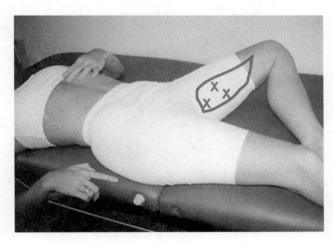

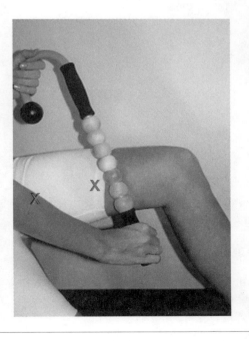

Check these TrPs:
Quadriceps group

Remember the rules for stretching and applying pressure

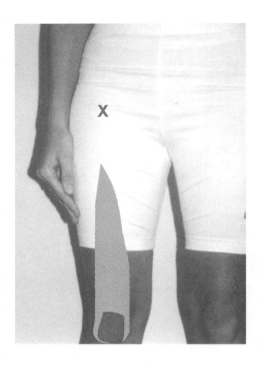

Related Dx's:

- Unexplained knee and thigh pain in children
- Hip joint disease
- Quadriceps tendonitis
- Jumper's knee

The Muscle:

The rectus femoris is one of the quadriceps muscle group that flexes the hip and   straightens the knee

Signs & Symptoms:

- Pain is felt deep in the knee
- Severe deep aching pain at night over the front of the lower thigh above the knee
- Sense of weakness

Causes:

- Acute: Sudden lengthening as in stepping into a hole, off curb or stumbling
- Direct trauma
- Skiing accident
- Chronic: Exercise program with deep knee bends
- Knee exercises (straightening the knee sitting with weight on ankle)
- Lifting 'correctly' with TrPs in soleus muscle
- Recovery from hip fracture
- Sitting with one leg tucked under the buttock
- Co-existing lumbar spine or hip joint disease
- Prolonged immobilization

Refer to Index, Legend, Figures, Glossary & Abbreviations

Management Tips:

- Use roller massage tool (photo below left)
- This is the only muscle in the quadriceps groups that crosses the hip and knee joint. Stretch by flexing the knee fully and then extending the hip; the back must be kept flat using a posterior tilt. (photo below right)

Preventing Recurrence:

- Reduce stress on muscle during lifting of heavy objects as in deep squat
- Use armrest to assist in standing from chair
- Avoid prolonged immobilization
- Avoid full hip flexion during sleep
- Avoid sitting with one foot under the buttock
- Correct flat foot

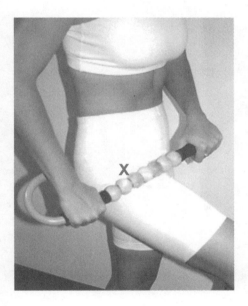

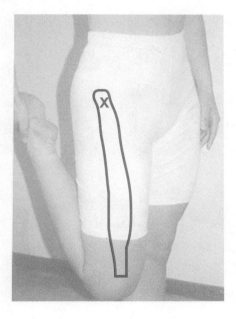

Check these TrPs:

Other quadriceps muscles
Hamstring group

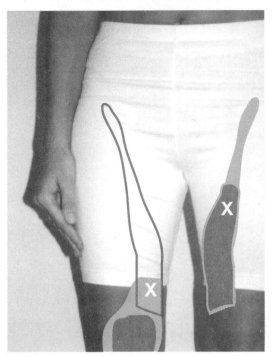

Related Dx's:

- Unexplained knee and thigh pain in children
- Hip joint disease
- Quadriceps tendonitis
- Jumper's knee
- 'Buckling knee muscle'

The Muscle:

The <u>vastus medialis oblique</u> (VMO) is one of the quadriceps muscles and extends the knee

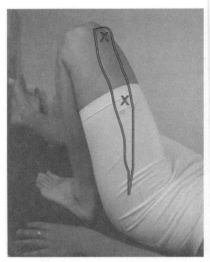

Signs & Symptoms:

- Toothlike pain deep in the knee joint
- Refers pain to anterior inside aspect of knee and up along inside of thigh
- Muscle may shut down causing the knee to give way
- Buckling more common on rough ground

Causes:

- Excessive flat foot
- Direct trauma to knee (i.e., hitting dashboard during car accident)
- Prolonged kneeling on hard surfaces
- Strenuous athletic activity such as jogging, skiing, football, basketball and soccer
- Co-existing lumbar spine or hip joint disease
- Shut down of muscle in shorter leg
- Falls

Refer to Index, Legend, Figures, Glossary & Abbreviations

Management Tips:

- Massage tool to apply direct pressure on TrPs and roller for stripping massage (see Ch. 17)
- The stretch comes from stabilizing the hip in extension with the low back kept flat and then slowly bending the knee.   Placing the foot on a footstool will allow a prolonged hold (photo below left)
- Stretch can be done with hip in flexion
- Contract-relax technique used on the quadriceps group may increase relaxation and ROM (see Ch. 17)
- Slight changes in the rotation kneeling on chair will change stretch from lateral to medial

Preventing Recurrence:

- Reduce stress on muscle during lifting of heavy objects; modify deep squat technique
- Use armrest to assist in standing from armchair
- Avoid sitting with one foot under the buttock
- Sitting up straight with legs out in front may aggravate symptoms
- Correct abnormal foot pronation
- Avoid prolonged immobilization
- Avoid full hip flexion during sleep

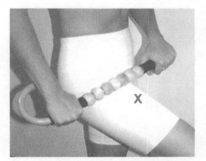

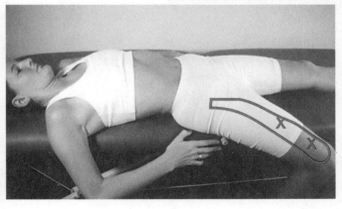

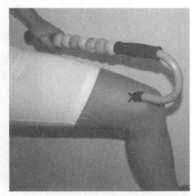

Check these TrPs:
Other quadriceps muscles
Hamstring group
Pectineus

Remember the rules for stretching and applying pressure

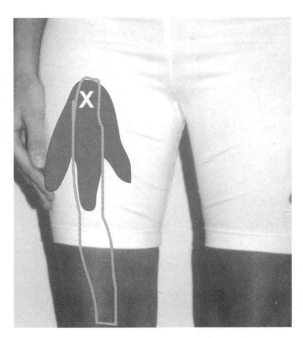

Related Dx's:

- Unexplained knee and thigh pain in children
- Hip joint disease
- Quadriceps tendonitis
- Jumper's knee

The Muscle:

The <u>vastus intermedius</u> of the quadriceps group assists in straightening the knee

Signs & Symptoms:

- Difficulty fully extending the knee
- After placing involved leg up on next step, cannot straighten knee
- Will limp after arising from a chair

Causes:

- <u>Acute</u>: Sudden lengthening as in stepping off curb into a hole or stumbling
- Direct trauma
- Skiing accident
- <u>Chronic:</u> Exercise program with deep knee bends
- Knee exercises (knee extension while sitting) with weight on ankle
- Lifting "correctly" with trigger points in soleus
- Recovery from hip fracture
- Sitting with one leg tucked under buttocks
- Prolonged immobilization
- Co-existing lumbar spine or hip disease

Refer to Index, Legend, Figures, Glossary & Abbreviations

Management Tips:

- Use roller tool for deep massage (photo below left, Ch. 17 for stripping technique)
- Stretch can be done with hip straight and low back stabilized or with hip flexed; the knee should be bent slowly. (photo below right)
- Contract-relax techniques can be used to get greater relaxation of the muscle (Ch. 17)

Preventing Recurrence:

- Reduce stress on muscle during lifting of heavy objects as in deep squat
- Use armrest to assist in standing from chair
- Avoid sitting with one foot under the buttock
- Avoid sitting up straight with legs out front
- Avoid prolonged immobilization
- Avoid full hip flexion during sleep
- Corrrect abnormal foot pronation

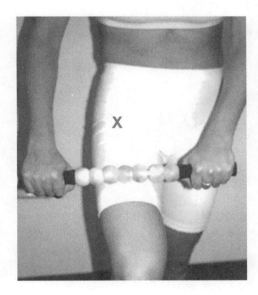
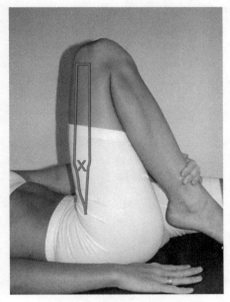

Check these TrPs:

Other quadriceps
Hamstring group

Remember the rules for stretching and applying pressure

135

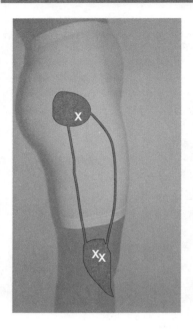

Related Dx's:

- Stuck patella
- Hip joint disease
- Iliotibial band syndrome

The Muscle:

The vastus lateralis oblique (VLO) assists in knee extension

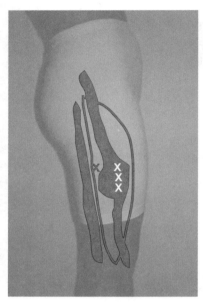

Signs & Symptoms:

- Lateral thigh pain from pelvis and greater trochanter to outside aspect of knee
- Pain from deep TrPs may 'explode' up and down thigh
- Pain around outside edge of knee
- Cluster of TrPs in mid-thigh causes severe pain over entire length of lateral thigh and up to crest of pelvis

Causes:

- Pain increased with walking
- Knee joint may be 'locked' making walking difficult or impossible
- Sudden overload, as in skiing
- Direct trauma, such as a fall, hitting the outer aspect of thigh
- In chronic low back pain, TrPs activated by poor gluteal stabilization of the hips/pelvis
- SI dysfunction may contribute to overuse
- Lying on involved side disturbs sleep
- Overuse due to postural dysfunction

Refer to Index, Legend, Figures, Glossary & Abbreviations

Management Tips:

- Use roller and work into deep massage (photo below right) or use direct pressure on points (photo bottom)
- Lie on involved side, placing tennis ball under TrP cluster
- Extreme sensitivity may benefit from low speed vibration
- Stretch by fulling flexing knee and holding, as in photo below left

Preventing Recurrence:

- Use armrest to assist in standing from chair
- Avoid full knee flexion during sleep
- Correct abnormal foot pronation
- Reduce stress on muscle during lifting of heavy objects; modify deep squat technique
- Sitting up straight with legs out front on ottoman may aggravate symptoms

- Avoid prolonged immobilization
- Avoid sitting with foot under buttock

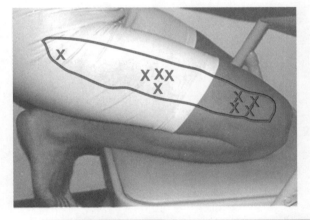

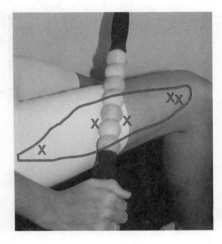

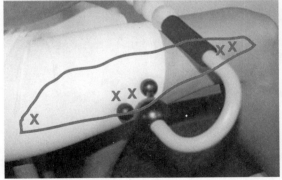

Check these TrPs:

Other quadriceps muscles
Hamstring group
Tensor fascia latae

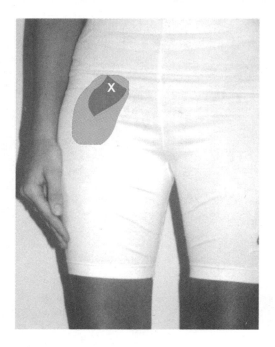

Related Dx's:

- Hip joint disease
- Pubic stress syndrome
- Fracture of the neck of the femur

The Muscle:

The pectineus muscle adducts and flexes the thigh

Signs & Symptoms:

- Pain is described as being deep in the groin
- Hip abduction may be limited

Causes:

- Acute: Tripping and/or falling
- Sudden, vigorous hip adduction-flexion movement, as in gymnastic exercises
- Chronic:
- Horseback riding
- Pain increased with weight bearing activity that abducts the thigh
- Leg length imbalance

Refer to Index, Legend, Figures, Glossary & Abbreviations

Management Tips:

- Pressure must be applied cautiously in center of groin (photo below left, top)

Preventing Recurrence:

- Correct leg length imbalance
- Avoid sitting in marked hip flexion
- Sleeping on uninvolved side, use pillow between knees and ankles to prevent shortening of the involved muscle
- Avoid sitting with legs crossed

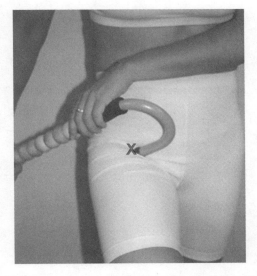

While doing these stretches it is critical that the back be kept flat. Doing a pelvic tilt by tightening the lower abdominal muscles will help keep the back flat. Pain should not be experienced in the low back with this stretch.

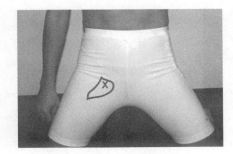

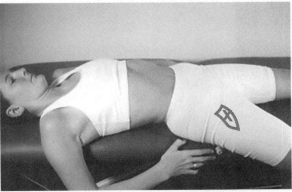

Check these TrPs:

Iliopsoas
Hip Adductors

Remember the rules for stretching and applying pressure

Anterior

Anterior tibialis

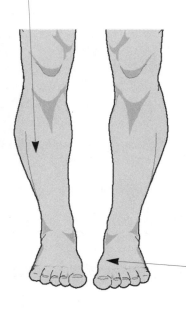

Posterior

Gastrocnemius
Soleus (deeper)
Tibialis posterior
(deepest)
Long toe flexors

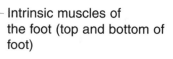

Intrinsic muscles of
the foot (top and bottom of
foot)

Lateral

Peroneus longus
Peroneus brevis (under longus)
Peroneus tertius
Long toe extensors

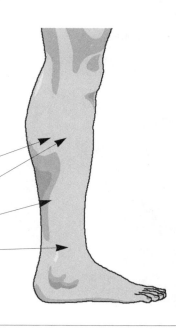

Chapter 10

Calf & Foot Pain

Pain in the calf or foot may have an elusive history of creating problems in many other areas of the body. One of the common themes throughout this book is the problem of Morton's foot syndrome, a structural foot problem described later in this chapter. When asking people what comes to mind when they think about pain in the foot and calf, common responses include flat feet or fallen arches, night cramps, shin splints, old ankle sprains or bunions. Many of these problems may have a history of muscle dysfunction long before they become painful enough to attract attention.

There are several TrPs in the pelvis or low back that refer pain to the foot or calf. One must always recognize the possibility that the cause comes from an area far from the site of the pain. Looking for the cause where the pain is may not result in a rapid resolution of the problem.

Pain Diagram

If you have not already done so, familarize yourself with the areas of the body where you most often experience your pain or symptoms by filling in the body diagram on the preceeding page, using the key on page 29. Mark the type of symptom you experience at each site and then look through the manual for similar patterns. After you have finished completing the diagram try answering questions in the checklist.

The Checklist

See what helps you in recognizing the things that contribute to increasing or decreasing your pain.

1.] What activities increase your pain? Are they all weight-bearing activities? Does the pain subside when you are off your feet?

2.] Do you have pain when walking and running?

3.] Do you have pain when biking (or some other activity)?

4.] Is your foot pain the same in all your shoes? What about when you go barefoot?

5.] Have you had ankle injuries that have resulted in an unstable ankle? You might know best by checking your range of motion of the ankle (how far you can move it actively) compared to your other foot or your friend's foot.

6.] Do you have what people generally refer to as "flat feet"? Are you developing a bunion (this is a bump on the outside of the big toe at its base)? Either of these may require orthotics or other intervention before the muscle pain can be effectively treated.

7.] If you are awakened by cramps in your calves at night, can you relate this to the level of activity you did that day, or any other factor that might provide clues as to its precipitating factor?

8.] Is the pain localized or diffuse?

Acute Trauma

Acute injuries such as fractures to the lower leg or ankle are common, and often result in prolonged casting for the fracture to heal. After the cast is removed, walking may be accomplished only with considerable limping, especially if the ankle range of motion is limited. Such a change in your gait pattern alters the work load on your leg muscles, causing some of them to work very hard and others to not work at all. In such a case, the muscles that overwork may be causing the pain. The same may be true after an ankle sprain. Although you may not have been casted, only taped or splinted, the changes in your gait pattern may have made one group of muscles work too hard at a job for which they are not accustomed.

Such injuries can lead to chronic muscle pain if the TrPs are not treated along with the scarring and range of motion. Direct damage to the muscles may not have occurred. It is the indirect damage as a result of how you have changed your gait that may be the primary source of your pain long after the fracture has healed.

Muscle overload can also cause acute pain. Running on a road's edge which is slanted can load one set of muscles excessively, as can running on uneven surfaces or with new shoes that are not broken in. The need to wear high heels after years of avoiding them may also cause sudden, acute muscle overload and pain.

Cumulative Trauma

The foot pain that develops over time may be the result of injuries that have not properly healed or feet that are not properly supported. Old ankle strains, with ligament damage, may not cause muscle pain in the calves for years. By then the need to try to stabilize the ankle joint to make up for lost ligaments begins to take its toll. You may not associate your current pain with old instability of the ankle unless you visit a practitioner skilled in evaluating this kind of problem.

The lack of proper foot support may also eventually give rise to foot and leg pain. How you place your foot on the ground when walking is critical to your overall function and movement, and doing it improperly several thousand times a day can amount to a painful muscle problem. Children, encouraged to wear trend setting shoes from a very early age have less of an opportunity to develop the muscles in their feet and calves than does the child allowed to run barefoot as much as possible.

The "growing pains" children experience may be the result of bones growing faster than muscle, pulling on the muscles and causing TrPs. Such pain may result in tendonitis and treatment such as spinting may provide some relief until the splint is removed. In such cases maintaining proper alignment of the feet with orthotics have often eliminated TrP pain in days and allowed the child to return to his/her normal levels of function. Ignoring such problems may seem prudent if you think the child will "outgrow" the problem, but often the muscle imbalances that develop follow the child into adulthood, with pain developing at a time when it may be much more difficult to alter the alignment dysfunction that has evolved over the years.

The mechanics of how you put your feet on the ground with each step you take is critical in how your entire body responds to gravity and the forces imposed by carrying, working and running. Trigger points may develop because the mechanics are poor, or they may be the cause of the mechanical faults that develop. Paying attention to the feet is a critical factor in maintaining good fitness habits.

Chronic Foot Pain

There are several chronic problems that can be examined for potential trigger points. These include problems attributed to plantar faciitis, shin splints, and achilles tendonitis. Examination of related TrPs might yield very promising results and rapidly increased function.

Keep in mind that prolonged limping or favoring of a painful foot may result in muscle pain in other areas. Differences in leg length that are either structural or functional may have contributed to mechanical foot problems in only one foot. Leveling the leg length requires careful determination of the functional or structural origin of the leg length difference. Orthotics that place the foot in proper alignment may cause an increase in pain if TrPs have developed prior to the use of the orthotics. The orthotics may not be the problem, and comfort may easily follow proper treatment of the muscle pain. Foot pain need not be accepted or expected and good problem-solving may yield unexpected results.

The Morton's Foot

The structure of the weight-bearing foot, if compromised, will resist successful treatment of the muscle pain if not corrected. In the case of the Morton foot, with a long second toe in relation to a short first metatarsal, years of walking with an adaptive gait pattern may take its toll on bone alignment and muscle. There is a normal weight bearing pattern during gait that may not be possible with a Morton foot structure, and changes in weight bearing can have an effect on the knee, hip, low back and even upper body areas. Combined with a bunion and abnormally pronated feet, significant muscle pain can develop and persist. A thorough evaluation of not only the foot, but your entire gait pattern is essential in reversing the effects of structural foot changes.

On Using the Section

Starting "from the bottom up" is not a bad way to look at any problem. In particular, foot, leg and pelvic problems often contribute to the perpetuation of pain in the low back, scapular area and neck. For good posture and function, start with good habits of foot mechanics and keep the feet fit. Looking through this section may give you clues as to how other problems have been perpetuated for long periods of time in spite of good, direct intervention. For good overall fitness, start at the feet and work your way up.

Figure 18

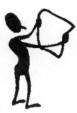

Chronic Pain as a Life Stresser

1. The person in pain usually becomes irritable, tolerating small hassles less easily, and frequently seeming to get angry wihout reason.

2. They may experience problems with sleeping, or getting restful sleep. Sleep deprivation contributes to a poor ability to cope with small hassles and aggravates pain.

3. Household chores may become a problem, and may lead to expec tations that someone else will do chores for them.

4. The patient with chronic pain often finds their job becomes painful and difficult, even if the job was not the original cause of the mus cle pain.

5. Pain throughout the workday may result in loss of productivity, higher risk of injury due to fatigue and lack of attention, and changes in one's relationship with coworkers and supervisors.

6. Finally, social activities may be curtailed. This may develop into isolation from the support of family and friends that is an important component to staying healthy.

7. In short, people with chronic pain are seldom fun to be around, nor do they often have fun.

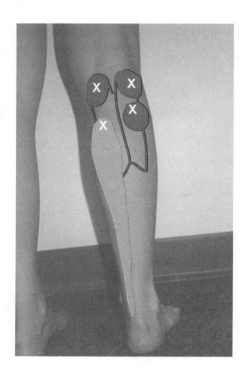

Related Dx's:

- Night leg cramps
- S1 nerve compression
- "Growing pains"
- Posterior compartment syndrome
- Phlebitis (blood clot)
- Achilles tendonitis
- Post-laminectomy syndrome

The Muscle: The gastrocnemius muscle is in the back of the calf, extending from just above the knee to the calcaneus. It plantar flexes the foot

Signs & Symptoms:

- Pain in the calf
- Leg cramps
- Pain behind the knee in activities requiring effort from the calf muscles, as in climbing, walking on uneven surfaces
- Partial tear ("Tennis leg")
- Pain in the arch of the foot

Causes:

- Long socks with tight elastic at the top
- Impaired circulation
- Chair too high for person; feet do not reach floor

Refer to Index, Legend, Figures, Glossary & Abbreviations

Management tips:

- It is critical that the gastrocnemius stretch be performed with the foot properly at a right angle to the wall, or the foot turned in slightly, with the heel kept down. If orthotics are gener ally worn, proper foot alignment might be better achieved with the shoes and orthotics on during the stretching
- Many get a better stretch using a slant board and doing both calves at the same time (photo below left)
- Stretching the gastrocnemius muscle and tightening the muscles that dorsiflex the foot before going to bed or if cramps occur during the night, is more helpful than walking after the cramp starts

Preventing Recurrence:

- Avoid shoes with high heels
- Use cruise control on car or take frequent breaks
- Avoid uneven, slanted surfaces when walking, running
- Eliminate tight elastic around calf
- Adjust firmness of accelerator pedal in car
- Excessive cooling while sitting i.e.,cold draft

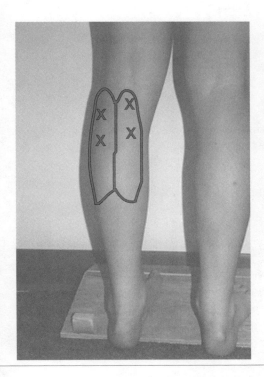
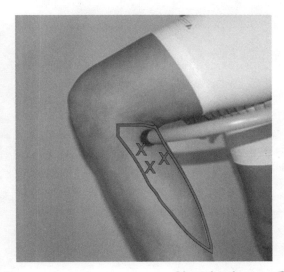

Check these TrPs:

Soleus
Hamstring
Tibialis posterior
Long toe flexors

Remember the rules for stretching and applying pressure

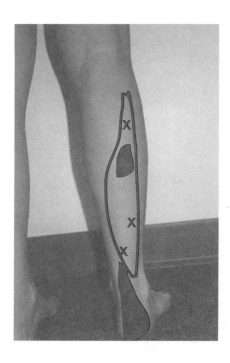

Related Dx's:

- Achilles tendinitis
- Rupture of the calf muscle
- Plantar fasciitis
- Thrombophlebitis
- Popliteal (Baker's) cyst
- Shin splints
- S1 nerve root compression

The Muscle:

The <u>soleus</u> muscle helps to stabilize the knee, provide ankle stability, plantar flexes and inverts the foot

Signs & Symptoms:

- Refers pain and tenderness mostly to the posterior aspect and bottom of the heel
- Pain is experienced near the insertion of the Achilles tendon into the heel bone
- Pain may be unbearable when weight is put on the heel as in standing
- The heel may ache at night
- Edema of the foot and ankle may be related to the trigger points above the knee
- Limited ankle ROM

Causes:

- Running
- Skiing or ice skating without adequate ankle support
- Walking on a surface that is smooth or slippery without adequate soles on shoes
- Hiking up a long steep hill

Refer to Index, Legend, Figures, Glossary & Abbreviations

Management Tips:

- A tennis ball used under the leg for direct compression of the TrPs
- The stretch is the same as the gastrocnemius stretch, but the knee is bent slightly (photo below left)
- Rollers to massage the muscle with the knee bent, or direct pressure on the TrPs (photo below right)

Preventing Recurrence:

- Avoid keeping the muscle in a shortened position for long periods
- Correction of leg length differences
- Avoid resting the the lower legs entirely on the calves, as in resting on a foot stool without support for the feet
- Support the feet at night so they are not plantarflexed
- Avoid high heeled shoes
- Pain walking upstairs may be reduced by placing the entire foot on the next higher step
- Keep the muscle lengthened with a good stretching program
- Stretch the muscle prior to running, tennis or other active sports

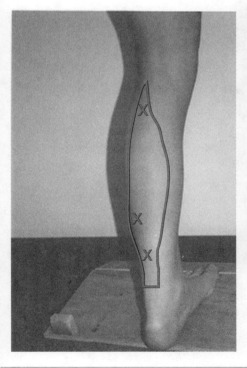
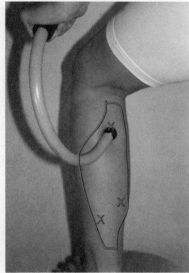

Check these TrPs:

Gastrocnemius
Posterior tibialis

Remember the rules for stretching and applying pressure

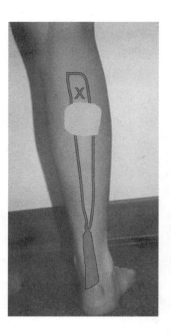

Related Dx's:

- Posterior compartment syndrome
- Shin splints
- Tarsal tunnel syndrome

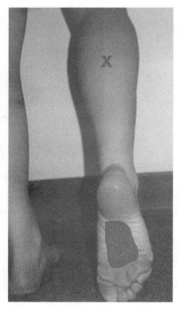

The Muscle:

The tibialis posterior muscle acts primarily to supinate the foot and to disperse weight bearing over the forefoot. The long toe flexors maintain balance and stability when weight is on the forefoot and during the mid and late stance phases of walking.

Signs & Symptoms:

- Pain over the Achilles tendon
- Pain in the sole fo the foot when running
- Pain in heel with walking
- Pain when walking or running on uneven ground

Causes:

- Running and jogging on surfaces that are uneven or slanted
- Footwear that is not worn well, lacking adequate support
- Hyperpronation of the foot due to poor mechanics, hypermobile joints, Morton foot structure

Refer to Index, Legend, Figures, Glossary & Abbreviations

Management Tips:

- Using a tennis ball placed under the leg in the long sitting position may provide effective ischemic compression
- Use a rolling pin or ball under the foot to loosen the foot joints
- Using rollers to provide a deep stroking motion (photo below right)

Preventing Recurrence:

- Run on smooth surfaces
- Corrective foot wear for Morton's foot structure; arch support for excessive pronation
- Avoidance of high heels
- Restoration of normal joint play if hypomobility is a problem
- Correction of muscle imbalances
- Ankle stabilization and proprioceptive training to increase efficiency of ankle musculature

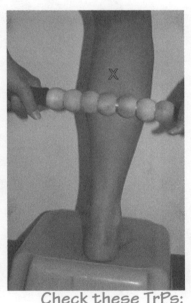

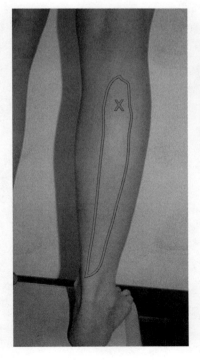

Stretch can be done on a slant board (left) or by stepping forward with the opposite foot, the involved foot behind and aligned with foot turned slightly inward, heel firmly on floor and knee bent slightly.

Check these TrPs:

Peroneal muscles
Flexor digitorum longus
Flexor hallucis longus
Toe extensors

Remember the rules for stretching and applying pressure

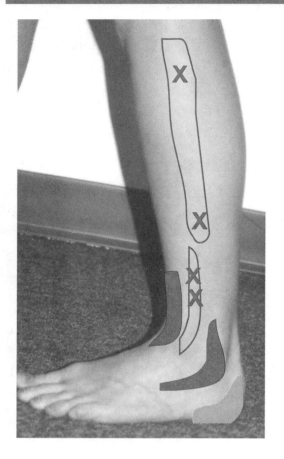

Related Dx's:

- Heel spurs
- Arthritis of the ankle

The Muscle: The <u>peroneus longus, brevis and tertius muscles</u> are located on the lateral side of the calf, extending from the fibula into the foot. These muscles control movement during standing and walking. The muscles will evert the foot when weight bearing

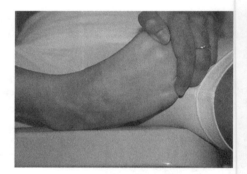

Signs & Symptoms:

- Weakness of the ankles
- Fall with inversion sprain in ankle
- Entrapment of peroneal nerve may cause pain & paresthesias of the top of the foot
- Numbness on top of first two toes (entrapment)

Causes:

- Immobilization, as in an ankle fracture
- Morton's foot structure
- Pronated foot problem
- Wearing high heels
- Leg length imbalance
- Crossing one leg over the other when sitting
- Ankle ligamentous instability laterally

Refer to Index, Legend, Figures, Glossary & Abbreviations

Management Tips:

- Contract relax techniques may make the muscle easier to stretch (see Ch. 17)
- This stretch should be felt along the lateral side of the calf, not at the ankle joint (photo opposite, right); ankle joint might be held to increase stretch to muscles
- Standing on slant board, inner aspect of foot should be slightly higher than outer edge (photo below left)

Preventing Recurrence:

- Correction of gait pattern from Morton's foot structure
- Elimination of high heel shoes
- Eliminate shoes with pointed toes, narrow toe box
- Avoid walking on slanted sidewalk or running on slanted surfaces

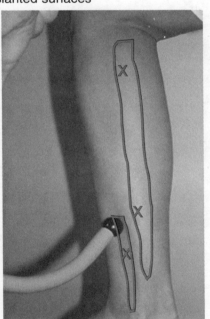

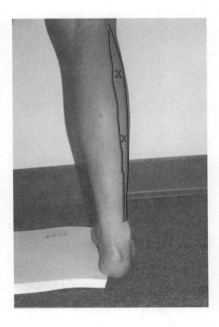

Check these TrPs:

Gluteus minimus

Remember the rules for stretching and applying pressure

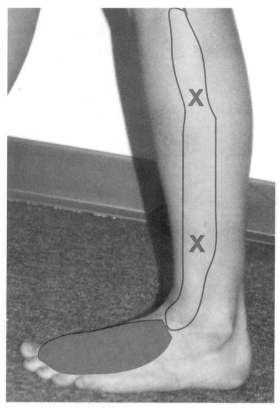

Related Dx's:

- Hammer toes caused by muscle imbalance

The Muscle:

The two muscles constituting the <u>long extensors of the toes</u> pull the toes up as well as controlling the foot slapping on the ground during heel strike. One muscle controls inversion, the other eversion of the foot during gait. The muscles are also active in controlling postural sway.

Signs & Symptoms:

- Pain over the top of the foot
- Night cramps in the long toe extensors
- "Foot pain"

Causes:

- Maintaining the muscle in a lengthened or shortened position, as in driving a car
- Wearing high heels
- A tight, shortened Achilles tendon
- Excessive jogging or running
- Stress fracture of the tibia or fibula
- Immobilization of the ankle after a fracture or sprain

Refer to Index, Legend, Figures, Glossary & Abbreviations

Management Tips:

- Someone with arthritis or instability in the ankle or knee might not want to perform this exercise, seated on the leg with the foot fully planter flexed (photo below right)
- Roller or stripping massage (see Ch. 17)

Preventing Recurrences:

- Correction of hypomobility in the joints of the foot
- Appropriate support for hypermobile joints in the foot
- Place car accelerator pedal in a more neutral position
- Avoidance of high heels
- Avoid running or jogging temporarily, then resume with proper foot support
- Support the ankle during sleep to avoid extreme plantarflexion

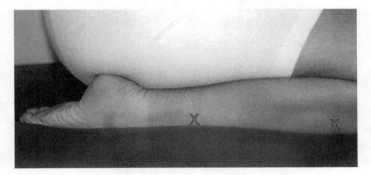

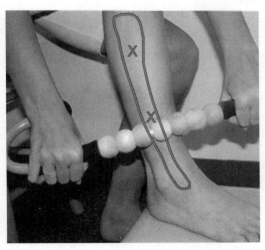

Check these TrPs:

Peroneal muscles
Tibialis anterior

Remember the rules for stretching and applying pressure

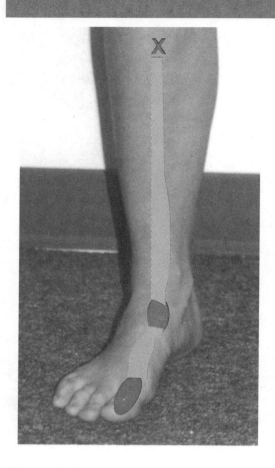

Related Dx's:

- Anterior compartment syndrome
- Shin splints
- L5 nerve root compression
- Rupture of anterior tibialis tendon

The Muscle: The <u>anterior tibialis</u> muscle dorsiflexes and supinates the foot. It also assists in maintaining standing balance. Prevents slapping of the foot down during walking.

Signs & Symptoms:

- Pain in big toe and front of ankle
- Pain moving ankle
- Dragging of the toes or ankle weakness
- Tripping or falling due to ankle weakness

Causes:

- Acute trauma
- Walking on rough ground
- Repetitive overuse
- Chronic tightness of muscles in the calf
- Morton's foot structure

- Ankle sprain
- Catching the toe on something during gait
- May follow anterior compartment syndrome

Refer to Index, Legend, Figures, Glossary & Abbreviations

Management Tips:

- Use of slow, deep stripping massage will assist deactivation of TrPs (see Ch. 17)
- Someone with arthritis or instability in the ankle or knee might not want to perform this exercise, seated on the leg, knee fully bend and foot plantarflexed (photo below right)

Preventing Recurrence:

- Correction of mechanical problems during gait, including Morton's foot structure
- Reduction in walking on uneven ground
- Maintaining the foot in a neutral position at night
- Strengthening program

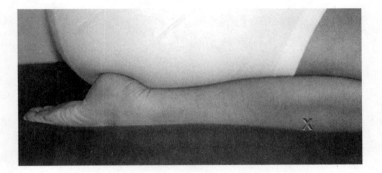

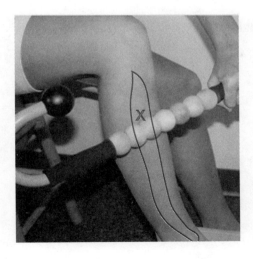

Check these TrPs:

Peroneus longus

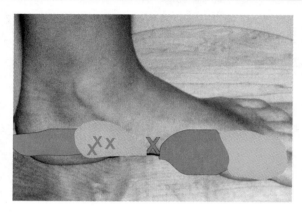

Related Dx's:

- Plantar faciitis
- Avulsion fracture of muscle attachment
- Sesamoid bone injury
- Other MPS

The Muscles:

The muscles that are <u>intrinsic to the foot</u> are mostly on the bottom of the foot, supporting the arch or flexing the toes. The muscles act to move the toes, and stabilize the foot during stance and gait.

Signs & Symptoms:

- The specific muscle determines the area of localized foot pain
- Deep, aching pain at rest
- Pain on bottom of heel
- Impaired walking due to pain
- May not tolerate orthotics until TrPs treated

Causes:

- Painful gait
- Hypermobile foot with excessive inversion or eversion
- Limited or hypermobile movement of any portion of the foot
- Morton's foot structure
- Sense of numbness of the foot, or swelling of the foot (when swelling is not present)
- Muscle imbalances and joint dysfunction

Refer to Index, Legend, Figures, Glossary & Abbreviations

Management Tips:

- Use rolling pin, golf balls, tennis balls to roll on the arch of the foot
- Small hand held device on the top of the foot (photo below right)

Preventing Recurrence:

- Proper foot wear with adequate support
- Restoration of normal foot flexibility with proper muscle length and joint motion

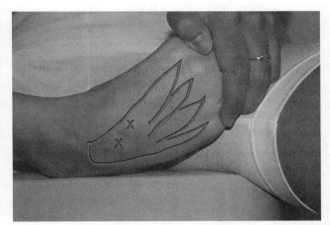

Strain on the outside of the ankle joint should be avoided during this stretch. Stabilize the ankle with the other hand.

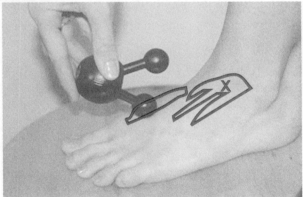

Check these TrPs:

Other TrPs in the foot

Remember the rules for stretching and applying pressure

Chapter 11

Muscles not covered in Other Sections

Muscles of the Face

Some of the muscles of the front of the neck, within the mouth and surrounding the eye have not been covered in the usual format. These muscles present unusual problems in terms of treatment and the assistance of a therapist well trained in treating these muscles would be appropriate.

These muscles may contribute to symptoms for TMJ (jaw) pain, headaches, difficulty swallowing, pain in several of the teeth and pain around the face, neck and under the ear.

Muscles within the orbit of the eyes are treated by some practitioners for symptoms related to focusing and synchonicity of eye movement to pain about the orbit. Be sure that the health care professional you choose has expertise in this area.

Muscles of Anterior Neck

These muscles, like those in the face, eye and mouth area, are difficult for individuals to do themselves. The muscles are important if you have been involved in motor vehicle accidents or have had neck surgery. Please consult a health care professional to evaluate the possible need for soft tissue work in this area.

Muscles in the Hands

There are many small muscles in the hands that have not been covered in depth in this book. Many of these would benefit from treatment of TrPs, and with the assistance of a health care professional to evaluate your needs, you may be able to do many of these yourself. These muscles are best evaluated along with the muscles in the forearms and the neck.

Muscles of the Pelvic Floor

There are a number of muscles that are categorized by their function, i.e., holding the pelvic floor contents. They are in effect a sling for lower abdominal contents. TrPs in these muscles may contribute to functional problems, i.e., incontinence or pain syndromes. There are often misdiagnoses with such problems as coccygodynia, endometriosis, prostatitis. Muscles adjacent to the pelvic floor, such as the glutei, adductors and rectus abdominis are often an integral part of the problem.

These TrPs are difficult to reach and just a few health care professionals have become skilled at working directly on pelvic floor muscles. Training and muscle re-education of these muscles may include direct pressure techniques on the muscles, biofeedback and muscle stimulation to the pelvic floor muscles. A combination of these may be more effective than a single technique. The comfort level of the patient measured with internal sensors (biofeedback) and digital pressure, must be considered at all times.

In Summary

The nature of MPS is elusive and often intermittent in nature, making the location of the primary problem more difficult. Changes occur in central pain processing. When a problem is chronic, subtle changes in these referral patterns may make it even more difficult for the TrPs responsible for a particular symptom to be found. A careful history, followed by a thorough physical exam is often necessary to determine where treatment should be initiated to provide the best overall results. Often, proper examination can be followed by instruction in home programs and development of a self management program. Some TrPs are just difficult for the individual to treat without help. It is then important to focus on identification of the factors that exacerbate those TrPs in a given individual so that prevention or rapid intervention when necessary can be accomplished without complex myofascial problems developing.

Chapter 12

Muscle Pain other than Myofascial Trigger Points

While this book attempts to simplify the complex problems of identifying and treating TrPs I, as the author, do not mean to imply that TrPs are the only cause of muscle pain. The other causes may be localized problems related to tissue inflammation or tearing, and general muscle pain, the most specific of these diagnoses being fibromyalgia. While not all factors causing muscle pain can be included here, the importance of some of these other factors cannot be overlooked. They will be discussed briefly.

Some causes of muscle pain arise within the muscle. The TrP is a good example. Other muscle pain problems arise from injury or dysfunction outside the muscle and are manifested by pain in muscle. Careful evaluation to differentiate the source of the pain is critical in establishing the proper treatment intervention. This is best done by a professional skilled in assessment and treatment of muscle pain, postural imbalances and movement dysfunction.

Musculotendinous Junction (MTJ)

The MTJ represents the zone toward the end of a muscle where the muscle fibers attach to its tendon. In certain muscles, this transition zone seems especially prone to an inflammatory pain syndrome. Also characteristic of this zone, the muscle fibers may be stiffer within the taut band than in the belly of the muscle.

The MTJ is the region of the muscle where a muscle "strain" is most likely to occur. Eccentric work, i.e., work done by the muscle as it is getting longer, may increase the likelihood of injury in the MTJ area.

The muscle may also be more prone to strain when it is accustomed to moderate levels of activity in only a small segment of the full range of the muscle and the demand imposed on the muscle is only in a limited range. Muscle flexibility, the ability of the muscle to comfortably go through a full range, may be the more critical deterent to incurring muscle strain when demands on the muscle are limited.

A technique of massaging across the MTJ portion of the muscle is often helpful in reducing this pain. Rapid relief may follow one minute of cross fiber massage described in Chapter 16.. The location of some frequent sites of MTJ pain have been identified in this manual in the Management Tips sections. If such techniques do not yield at least immediate temporary relief, examination of this area by a health professional should be considered.

Insertion Pain

Pain at the muscle's insertion or fixation point is much like the pain at the MTJ zone, but occurs in the area of the tendon where it attaches to bone or ligaments. This "tendinitis" may be very localized and acute, or may be experienced as more diffuse throughout a portion of the muscle.

Insertion pain is often treated at the same time as TrPs are deactivated. The area of the muscle where the TrP is located is shortened, often described as a taut band or nodule. The shortening of muscle cell segments (sarcomeres) in the area of the TrP require that other sarcomeres lengthen to compensate. This lengthening often occurs near the attachment of the muscle to bone or the formation of the tendon. The chronic strain placed on this tissue may result in the insertion pain. The use of a cross fiber or transverse friction massage technique may be useful for this type of muscle pain.

Entrapments

An entrapment is a phenomenon occurring in soft tissue where one tissue (i.e., the nerve) is trapped or squeezed by surrounding tissue. Over time, this produces changes in the tissues and may reflect damage to the nerve. When a nerve is squeezed the ability of the nerve to function may be altered and muscles innervated by that nerve may be affected.

Muscles in spasm and muscles with TrPs may cause entrapment of a nerve or its branches. The sensation caused by the entrapment include sensations of burning, tingling or numbness. Rather than motor nerves to muscle being entrapped, sensory nerves to the skin may be the problem.

The entrapments may be postural, positional or due to secondary changes in muscle length and tension due to injury or TrPs. Compression may involve nerves and/or blood vessels, changing the symptom presentation from pain and numbness related to the nerve being compressed, and coldness or discoloration when the compression is vascular.

A few of the common entrapments include the scalene muscles in the neck, the pectoralis minor muscle in the front of the shoulder and the piriformis muscle deep in the buttocks. You can find TrP pages on these muscles in this manual.

With many varieties of the anatomical configuration of nerves and vessels, symptom presentation may vary from one individual to the next. While TrPs may contribute to the development of an entrapment, or develop subsequent to the nerve compression due to irritation, treatment of an entrapment syndrome may necessitate the advice of a qualified health care professional.

Radiculopathy

This term represents a specific type of nerve entrapment, generally involving a disc in the spine or narrowing of the neural foramen of the spinal nerve. The source of the pain comes from the area of the spine, not the muscle where it might be felt. While the pain and sensory changes are referred, the symptoms occur in a particular pattern related to the nerve root. The pain may be experienced as muscle pain but it originates from problems outside the muscle.

This type of referred pain and numbness may be accompanied by loss of muscle strength and may suggest a more serious problem. Such nerve root problems should always be ruled out if there is any question as to the source of symptoms.

Muscle Soreness related to Exercise

This type of muscle pain is generally referred to as delayed onset muscle soreness and is most common following exercise. It may be acutely felt at the MTJ but appears as a diffuse pain throughout the muscle. It is related to lengthening contractions of the muscle or fibers within a muscle.

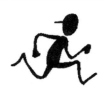

Figure 20

Hurt vs. Harm

Hurt: When you feel more pain after you do an activity - you may have sore muscles for awhile - but you have not caused any physical damage to yourself.

Harm: When you push yourself beyond your limits, and physical damage may occur. This is NOT often the case; being sore and hurting are much more often the case. Respect the restrictions you have been given.

The initiation of exercise starting with light exercise to protect against or reduce the post exercise soreness of later heavy bouts of exercise has been suggested. It has been reported to be more effective in some muscle groups than in others.

The evaluation of muscle soreness that arises from initiating an exercise program after long abstinence requires distinguishing "harmful" muscle pain versus "hurtful" muscle pain. The former may result from too heavy an exercise program without proper training or conditioning and may signal injury, while the latter is a discomfort expected after doing an activity that has not been done for a long period of time when the muscle is "out of shape." The ability to discriminate between "hurt" and "harm" is criticial to taking on new exercise or activity after a long period of being sedentary.

tic tests often come back negative, frustrating both physician and patient.

Fibromyalgia is defined as painful, predominantly involving muscles, and is the most com-

Fibromyalgia

A discussion of fibromyalgia would require a book itself. This book is not designed to make an intense effort to differentiate between myofascial pain syndrome with TrPs and fibromyalgia. As with MPS, diagnos- mon cause of chronic, widespread musculoskeletal pain. Fibromyalgia generally characterizes a diffuse muscle pain involving many

---

Figure 21

Myofascial Pain Syndrome vs. Fibromyaliga

Differences

TrPs	Fibromyalgia
1 female : 1 male	~ 7 females : 1 male
Regional pain	Widespread pain
Focal tenderness	General tenderness
Muscle feels tense	Feels soft & doughy
Reduced ROM	Hypermobile
Tigger point exam	Tender point exam
TrPs respond well to injection	TrPs (when present) respond poorly
20% also have fibromyalgia	72% also have active TrPs

(See References/Recommended Reading in Appendix C)

---

segments of the body and related to rapid and chronic fatigue in muscle after even brief exercise. Also commonly present are persistent fatigue, generalized morning stiffness, non-refreshing sleep and tender points. Other problems commonly seen as part of the syndrome include headaches, dysmenorrhea, sensitivity to cold, irritable bladder, restless legs, and complaints of weakness.

It is not uncommon, however, to have myofascial pain syndrome and TrPs coexist in someone with fibromyalgia. The MPS and TrPs may be localized and the result of an injury to only one body part. Such distinction is not always clear but may provide insight into why treatment of TrPs in an individual with fibromyalgia is often appropriate and necessary.

Chapter 13

Stress, Exercise and Myofascial Pain Syndrome

Lack of adequate exercise may increase the risk of developing muscle pain. Only recently has physical activity been seen as recreational activity, rather than a normal part of living. Several generations ago, the exercise that was obtained while one fed farm animals, worked in the fields all day, rode horseback or walked to and from school included sustained levels of cardiovascular workout greater than most recreational athletes obtain in an hour at the health club. Such activity was not balanced by total sedentary living, i.e., sitting at a desk, driving a car, or sitting with a TV remote control the rest of the day.

> Business travel often increases stresses. Find a way to continue some form of exercise program on the road.

Many of us see exercise as something we must find time to add into our workday, not as an integral part of it. Exercise presents time management problems as work encroaches on more and more leisure time for many people who see exercise as something they have to deliberately add to a day rather than being a part of it. A cardiovascular workout did not need to be squeezed into anyone's day and monitored for maximum time above "target heart rate" - it was the majority of an individual's day. When we are not exercising we are creating postural problems, not relaxing. The counterbalance to early 1990's life was sitting and relaxing in the evening, activity dictated by the light given off from the fire, a candle or lantern. Being sedentary was a minimal portion of the pioneer's day. In contrast, any exercise we do at the health club is a minimal part of our day, the rest spent sitting at a desk or performing the same task with minimal variation and not taking care of postural adaptation to such sedentary living.

The lack of exercise throughout the day also reduces our ability to blow off steam when we encounter a stressor. We tend to hold onto stress longer and pay a greater physiological price for having encountered the stressor. If we don't exercise that day, the stressors continue to have an impact on our life, perhaps for days. If exercise is the only stress management technique by which we deal with such stressors, it is dependent upon finding recreational time or time out from our daily activities. Often we perceive such activity with limited enjoyment, but necessary to maintain our weight, decrease risk of heart attack, etc.

Stress

The difference in our use of the flight or fight response can be seen with another, all too frequent example of how our stress has become so chronic. Think of yourself driving along a highway on your way to work in the morning. Rush hour traffic always annoys you, and the traffic seems slower than normal today. You are thinking you might be late to the meeting at 8:00, where you are expected to do the first presentation. You are also coordinating the meeting, and know that no one else will start the meeting if you are not present. All of a sudden, a car coming from the on ramp cuts sharply in front of you. You grab the steering wheel trying to get out of his way, and hope the car in the next lane is not too close. You lay on the horn, scream about the idiocy of the world and try to keep from running your car into the car that has just pulled out.

Minutes later you pull off your exit and into work. You are still fuming about the near miss. You enter your office and rush into the meeting. Along the way several people hear about the near miss, and also notice the anger in your voice and your body. Your body language when you walk into the meeting is "don't mess with me". Your day continues to be very stressful and when you get settled back into the car to drive home you think again about the driver from that morning. You might even glance about several times, thinking you might spot them. You were late getting out of the office and have to deal with Friday traffic drivers heading north for their cabins, so it takes longer to get home. You are planning to go out to eat with a friend and the only way you can be on time is to skip the health club.

Does this sound like a healthy response to that very short-lived stressor? Who, in the long run, is paying a greater price for that person pulling out in front of you? That person who almost cut you off has no awareness he did anything to upset you, went about his business and is probably enjoying some recreational exercise. You on the other hand, are still reliving the experience, and so is your body.

> Flexibility & aerobic exercise are key elements in keeping myofascial TrPs under control.

Exercise as Relaxation

When exercise, which is generally considered recreational in our culture, is the only means of relaxing, the body has an opportunity to burn off some of that stress. We usually feel better after we have finished the exercise program. However, our body does not get to do any repair work, or rebalancing. It needs some down time to reduce the effects of poor sitting posture, carrying a heavy briefcase or bookbag over the shoulder for hours, sitting with a stiff back and taking the elevators rather than the stairs. Not to mention reducing the effects of that driver that cut you off. We generally don't find a lot of time to come home, sit and listen to music and just relax for any length of time. Often the music becomes noisy background, adding subtle stress to our body rather than reducing it. We move on through the evening, get to our office work late, then finally have to do a few household chores and head for bed later than normal. Once again, we might wrestle with that driver, or the impact our anger had on the meeting that morning, and we resolve to get some exercise in the coming days. But where to find the time? Having friends who also work out is one option; it is easier to keep an appointment with someone else than with ourselves, and having someone to exercise with often makes the time pass more quickly.

Fatigue & Myofascial Pain Syndrome

Individuals with fibromyalgia have been identified as having low endurance levels with exercise or physical activity. While the fatigue has been shown to be less of a generalized problem in people with MPS, there is a tendency for muscles with latent TrPs to tire more rapidly than muscles without latent TrPs and be susceptible to reactivation of the TrPs with fatigue or states of chronic stress. Pacing often becomes critical in completing long, physically-demanding tasks. If the MPS is localized to only one or two muscles, it is unlikely the fatigue will be noticed easily. If latent TrPs exist in a number of muscle groups, then the change in movement that may precede the reactivation of TrPs may provide some warning to take a break. For many, the same amount of physical work can be accomplished - the trick is to be able to stop, taking a break to stretch or treat a TrP, and then get back to the task.

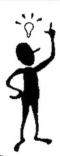

Figure 22

A Stress Checklist

PHYSICAL

___stomach upsets
___grinding teeth
___racing heart
___inability to sit still
___frequent colds
___difficulty sleeping
___increase/decrease in weight
___eating more when not hungry
___shopping to feel better
___wandering around aimlessly
___hives
___wanting to be alone - not typical
___unable to sit still

EMOTIONAL

___easily angered
___explode without reason
___crying easily
___down in the dumps
___cannot stop worrying
___don't laugh any more
___nothing feels good
___don't want to be around family, friends
___anxious
___poor concentration
___rapid changes in mood

Chapter 14

Chronic Postural Stress

Many of the activities that we engage in create an asymmetrical, or lopsided, loading of the muscles of our body. One activity that is rampant in our culture is the carrying of bookbags, purses and soft sided briefcases over one shoulder. The student who starts carrying that bookbag to elementary school is going to have some symptoms before he gets through high school. Symptoms might be subtle, occasional and not worth addressing, but those muscle imbalances, and adaptive changes will have an impact should an injury occur.

Other cultures have resolved such carrying problems by learning to carry items on the head, or using yokes over the shoulder. Sounds funny and you would never do such a thing because it is not the in thing to do, right? Those people were doing something with sound, basic ergonomic principles, i.e., balanced the load, and reducing a number of forces on the spine and shoulder. That one sided bookbag habit or large purse will often lead to TrPs and pain. The points you might want to explore include the Trapezius, Levator scapulae and Serratus posterior superior. Headaches arise from the lower trapezius TrPs, neck pain from the levator scapulae muscle.

Old Injuries

Old injuries also have an impact on the development of MPS and TrPs. Perhaps one of the most common is the whiplash that results from a motor vehicle accident. Several mechanisms may later trigger headaches after all the neck problems seem to have resolved. One is from the muscle activity in the neck becoming lopsided, or asymmetrical. This can happen at the time of the accident, and can easily be treated at that time. However, if muscle length and muscle recruitment patterns are not corrected, TrPs in the SCM may again create headache problems that seem unrelated to the old car accident. Other muscles, deeper in the neck, also become shortened and tight or stretched out. They may be anterior, lateral or posterior neck muscles. When the lateral neck muscles (the scalenes) or the pectoralis minor muscle shorten and tighten, there may evolve symptoms that go down into the hands that might be carpal tunnel syndrome. While actual carpal tunnel syndrome may develop in someone who has had a motor vehicle accident and may be entirely unrelated, these symptoms from the scalenes can easily be treated if caught early. While TrPs in these muscles do not cause headaches in and of themselves, they generally exist with the SCM TrPs, which do result in headache symptoms. Old injuries may mean that certain muscles are more vulnerable to reactivation of latent TrPs from chores or sports, that require little effort.

Postural Imbalances & Positional Stresses

Postural imbalances can lead to muscle pain and TrPs. These postural problems may be structural or functional. Both may need to be addressed. The structural problem may be a leg length imbalance created by a fractured leg when a child, or one leg being shorter than the other after an individual completes the growth period. When the upper arms are shorter proportionally than they should be, they do not reach the armrests on most chairs and a more forward posture is required to rest them on a desk, creating other postural challenges. Leg length imbalances, for example, cause the muscles of the neck to work harder to keep the eyes level. The shoulder on one side may normally be higher, but balance is dependent upon the head working to adjust, creating a level visual plane. This puts a lot of stress on one of the neck muscles, and headaches from this extra work load is common. The muscle, known as the SCM, must be examined and treated carefully, as triggering a headache or a brief dizzy

Figure 23

Postural Stresses

The types of stress that may be imposed by structural malalignment may include, but not be limited to:

1) Leg length imbalance	Old fracture, old knee injury
2) Differences in proportions within body segments	Short upper arms
3) Environmental stress	Mismatch of furniture & body size
4) Work station design	Improper height of monitor
5) Overuse of muscles due to task demands	Static job with repetitive overuse of one joint or limb

spell is not uncommon.

The issue of both leg length imbalance and the structural fault mentioned often in this manual, Morton's foot syndrome, have been discussed separately in another section of this chapter. It is important to become aware of factors that increase muscle pain. These may be as simple as sitting in a chair that does not fit well, such as with arm rests that are too low. This may not be a problem if you only sit in the chair when waiting briefly for an appointment, but may be a major factor if it is the chair that you sit in at work, or the majority of the time in your home. Chairs are built for a "standard" size, a one size fits all approach. People vary not only in height and width, but in the relative lengths of body segments. Individuals of normal height may find their upper arms are short, requiring that they lean to one side to rest their elbow on the armrest. This type of mis-fit between body and chair places a strain on muscles, joints and soft tissues. If someone already has muscle pain, such stress will tend to increase or perpetuate the pain.

Our bodies were designed for a wide variety of movement and with the expectation that

The squirming of youngsters the first months of school might serve as a good reminder of what our bodies are designed to do - move!

a wide variety of movement would be performed. The more sedentary we become, restricting not only variation in joint range of motion and muscle length opportunities but limiting variety for our muscles to perform a wide range of tasks. These factors increase the risk for injury when we do perform novel tasks. The soreness that is often associated with the "weekend warrior" who only plays tennis on weekends, or who thinks they can cut several cords of firewood in one day after sitting at a desk for five long workdays may reflect such occasional changes in activity. Those individuals who sit and perform repetitive tasks, day after day, changing their muscle tension little, changing the task demand seldom, may be putting the greatest stress on their body. Chapter 15 has been dedicated to a discussion of repetitive strain injury (RSI).

Over the years of disciplining ourselves to sit for long hours, the signals from our body that we are uncomfortable may not even reach consciousness. We accept the chair and our sitting long after our muscles have asked to move about. Combine that with the performance of tasks such as typing, assembly work or other repetitive jobs and we have muscles that are asked to perform only one task, at only one muscle length, with unending repetition and little variation. Early messages of pain and fatigue are squelched in the need to "get the job done" and overuse with muscle pain becomes the presenting problem. It is a problem because in the late stages, individuals are finding recovery to be an elusive goal and one which places enormous challenges upon one's lifestyle.

Muscle pain may be the first, or primary symptom, or it may reflect a joint dysfunction that has long been ignored. Dysfunction in the sacroiliac joint (or SI joint) is often overlooked for years, leading to chronic low back pain, neck and shoulder pain, and even migraine headaches. When the foundation of what balances the body, i.e., the pelvis, is not aligned correctly the rest of the body must struggle constantly to keep itself above the lopsided foundation. The result is not a body that gets to rest in a balanced posture, but one which constantly struggles to portray itself as balanced, often at great cost in terms of muscle work, muscle adaptation of length and tension, and muscle pain.

The forward head posture seen so often in people who are mostly sedentary and have poor muscle balance and muscle tone requires that muscles in the back of the neck work continuously to hold "the bowling ball from falling off its ledge." In fact, the head weighs about as much as a bowling ball (12 pounds) and the lack of a balanced position above the neck and shoulders leads to a lot of work and postural stress. Muscles, instead of getting a rest when appearing inactive, are working overtime to keep the head on the neck and there is no rest, even when the person is weary. Some muscles are overstretched, others shortened. Add to such postural stress a minor motor vehicle accident and you have an individual headed for chronic pain.

Postural and positional stresses of any kind bear correction. If you have a fixed amount of energy to spend in one day, would you rather spend it all just trying to hold yourself up against the forces of gravity? Or would you rather have some of that energy, like a credit card out of debt, to spend on social events, sports, and pleasurable hobbies. Rather than coming home from work exhausted, wanting only to rest for the energy demands known to be waiting the next day, wouldn't you rather come home with surplus credit on that credit card, willing and able to be active? Even stresses imposed by high level

> Need help squirming at your desk at work? Sit on an air filled cushion shaped like the top of a ball and give your back muscles the workout they are looking for!

athletic competition, positive as it may be, can be a problem when the imbalances of some sports are not addressed, leaving a body strong, well developed in muscle bulk, but poorly able to fight the symmetrical forces of gravity.

Leg Length Imbalances

One of the more common arguments among the health professionals treating orthopedic problems is the importance, or lack of importance, of having a leg length imbalance. How much matters? It is common for me to work with chronic low back pain patients who have a leg length imbalance, determine whether it is structural or functional, correct the problem and see much of their pain and symptoms resolve. In a similar fashion, there are a group of individuals with migraine headaches who see marked improvement in their symptoms when long-standing leg length imbalances are corrected and neck muscle dysfunction and trigger points can be corrected. These individuals have been fighting for years to keep a head level on an uneven base of support.

An analogy might be helpful. Think about (or briefly try for yourself) putting on one flat shoe and one shoe with a high heel and walking around like that for several hours, weeks or even months. Do you think you might get pain in your body other than your feet? Such an imbalance puts tremendous stress on the low back, and the upper trunk muscles must also work harder. The head, following the lead of the pelvis would be severely tilted. In the effort to right itself, the body must ask some muscles to work very hard and others to stop doing their usual job. The result is a lot of muscle and joint stress.

How much of a leg length imbalance makes a difference? That question is hard to answer. Some professionals think that if you can't see it, it is not causing any harm. Others just don't think any leg length difference is important if you are not having pain. The problem is that by the time you do have pain, the work needed to change the muscle imbalances is much greater than it would have been if treated earlier.

How do you "fix" a leg length imbalance? First, a qualified health professional must determine if the leg length is structural or functional. A structural one is one for which there are permanent or unocrrectable changes. It might also be the result of a fracture in one of the leg bones, with the bone healing shorter than the

> Correcting postural malalignment that is chronic and involves more than one joint is often a lengthy process. It requires a team effort and patience to reverse long-standing dysfunction.

other leg. A functional leg length imbalance, on the other hand, is one which is a product of poor joint alignment or muscle imbalances within some area of the body, usually the hips, pelvis and low back. This type of leg length imbalance can be changed if the alignment is corrected and the muscles returned to their normal lengths. An individual with an SI problem, or back pain, may develop shortening of some muscles of the low back, hiking the hip, or altered alignment of the hip sockets which in effect changes the length of the legs.

There are very few occasions when a functional leg length imbalance should be treated with a lift in the shoe, in effect maintaining the malalignment of the joints and muscles. Treatment of TrPs, often found in the shortened muscles, is part of the overall treatment of functional leg length imbalances. The

dysfunction must first be accurately and correctly assessed, and then a treatment program designed to correct the faulty postural alignment. This includes shortening some tissue and lengthening other tissue. It means that some joint capsules will have to allow greater freedom of movement in a direction that has been narrowly contained. Correcting postural malalignment that is chronic and involves more than one joint is often a lengthy process. It is a team job, with the client doing much of the work and the health professional directing the movement changes.

When the leg length imbalance is structural, the structural imbalance should be corrected. This might be done with a lift inside the shoe if the difference is small, or a thicker sole built on the outside of the shoes if the imbalance is greater. Even with correction of the structural imbalance, especially one that is chronic, muscle and soft tissue changes must

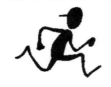

Figure 24

Signs of Leg Length Imbalance

1. Does one pant leg seem longer than the other?

2. Do you stand on one leg when waiting in line - it is always the same leg?

3. When you stand on one leg is the other leg out to the side, turned out?

Note: If standing level feels awful, put a 1/4" magazine under one foot and try again. If this feels more level, do not add a shoe lift without consulting a professional.

be taken into consideration. If the imbalance is 1/4 inch or more, the adjustment for correction should be gradual, adding a little to the lift each few weeks. It is not uncommon for this process to take months and those clients with chronic headaches or migraines will need to be especially careful.

Shoulder problems, even thoracic outlet syndrome, like headaches, may be traced to a leg length imbalance as one of the perpetuating factors in the dysfunction. A health care professional who is qualified to treat such problems should be able to evaluate postural problems for the impact they may be having on the your symptoms.

To return to the question of "how much leg length imbalance matters" the answer is that very little imbalance may be sufficient to create a persistent cycle of chronic pain once an injury has occurred. Small differences in leg length may have been present for many years, and usually are, before someone has an injury. The injury may be cumulative in nature, meaning that the years of stress and strain on the body from the imbalance has been a contributing factor to making someone vulnerable to an injury. After an injury the long-used compensatory, adaptive patterns can no longer be sustained without pain or other symptoms. A small, negligible leg length imbalance becomes a big problem for some muscles after they have been injured. The quadratus lumborum, a deep back muscle, is a good example.

Sustained pain from postural dysfunction is common and may often be a major contributing factor in chronic pain syndromes. The adaptive changes may have allowed an athlete to finish his last ten races, or a data entry operator to complete the 20 years she needed for her pension, but those changes have taken a toll on muscles, soft tissue and joints. Maintaining a healthy postural alignment is just as important as having good vision or bi-yearly dental check-ups. If you want to keep moving, have your body alignment checked at least as often as you do the alignment of your car.

The Morton's Foot: A Domino Effect

The Morton foot may be a ghost in the closet of some individuals who have had muscle pain for years. How many of you have examined your feet to better understand your low back pain? Or, have you considered how your feet hit the ground to understand your pain in the muscles of the neck and shoulders? The Morton's foot problem is characterized by a second toe that is longer than the first toe due to relative length differences of the metatarsal bones.

The classic description of what a Morton's foot syndrome may cause in the way of symptoms might include a list as diverse as low back pain, muscle pain in the thigh, knee, leg and foot. Such individuals may describe their foot problem, if they are aware of one at all, as one in which the ankles are weak and often sprained. The relatively long second toe changes the weight-bearing that occurs through the stance phase or walking,, and how the foot assists in the push-off as the next step begins. These changes in the force trajectory change the force and angle of the knee during stance as well as the alignment of the hip. The symptoms may become widespread, with TrPs contributing to the pain. The final clinical presentation, if not addressed, may mimic a lumbar disc problem, causing pain on the low back rather than on the foot.

The foot problem can be evaluated by an experienced health professional. The postural imbalances and symptom presentation may vary widely, and assistance may be needed to distinquish the multiple factors that can be influenced by a long second metatarsal. Correction of the foot mechanics with orthotics may exacerbate other muscle pain as the weight-bearing demands have changed. The addition of orthotics in an individual with a Morton's foot syndrome and muscle pain may be a lengthy procedure and one which generally needs pro-

> Studies have shown a high incidence of TMJ dysfunction often years after a motor vehicle accident. This may be only one of dozens of examples of how old injuries may be related to new problems.

fessional problem-solving until a new level of movement balance can be achieved.

Old Injuries: New Problems

Many of us sustain injuries throughout our lifetime. Many are injuries that we shake off due to youth, i.e., "children heal quickly" or we forget or are unaware of injuries won in the heat of battle, such as a high school basketball playoff game. Then there are the injuries that we acquire being a "weekend warrior" or carpenter for a day. These injuries often claim less glory than those of our youth and their subsequent aches and pain are shrugged off as an expected part of aging. However, each or all of these injuries may create subtle trouble, causing slight changes in our biomechanics, the muscles that are used for activities, or strain on a joint. Add on a few more injuries, and the mechanics of movement become even more dis-ordered. These changes in movement may not cause us any real problems. They may be the aches we wake up with in the morning but which are gone by the time we leave for work, or they may be the fatigue we experience when we are driving toward the gym after work. They can affect the intensity or length of our workout.

Subtle Muscle Compensation

Subtle muscle compensation is very common. While we may first think that anyone who is not in sufficient pain to be a "patient" is moving normally, many people are compensating on a subtle level. This compensation is evident in the therapists I train, who measure muscle dysfunction using multiple channels of surface EMG. This technique is designed to evaluate muscle dysfunction in patients who have chronic pain. Examination of hundreds of practicing health professionals, mostly physical and occupational therapists, demonstrate clearly that subtle muscle dysfunction is present in most people, whether they are currently having pain or not. Many of these therapists, when seeing the muscle dysfunction, can relate it to an old injury or to occasional soreness at the end of the day, or after sport activities. The muscle dysfunction has characteristics that differ from the dysfunction seen in patients in the extent and severity of the dis-ordered muscle activity. But it is present, as if a portent of what might be to come.

Such changes in movement create a faulty foundation on which movement continues for many more years. We all know that individuals who have severe movement problems, such as severe polio, cerebral palsy or a stroke, generally move less, and are involved in sporting leisure activities less than those without these and other movement disorders. Their limitation is more obvious and their total activity at the end of a day more limited.

We seldom expect an individual who has suffered a stroke to complete three sets of tennis, yet someone with subtle movement dysfunction may be just as reluctant to play tennis or another sport. They may have less understanding of why they are reluctant, but hesitate and feel they would rather participate in more casual activity. These faulty foundations create the possibility of greater problems if more injuries follow. Such subtle injuries may cause a faulty mechanical problem that could portent potential disaster if that same individual were to sustain only a certain kind of injury. This might be like the architecture of a home that makes it vulnerable to damage if a tornado where to hit from only one certain direction.

Each of our faulty foundations may make us vulnerable for only one injury, and many of us are never exposed to that one potential disaster of a mechanical insult. But for a few, that injury happens, and recovery becomes a nightmare. They have come back from so many injuries,

> Old injuries, long forgotten, may result in simple new problems becoming chronic symptom generators. Old injuries do come back to haunt us.

they often wonder why they cannot come back from this, often "minor" injury. They are unaware that this injury creates a domino effect with other injuries and dis-ordered movement, recovery suddenly miles away and the road-blocks poorly understood. For many, this is a set up for chronic pain, a lengthy recovery that seems destined to fail time and again despite one's best efforts. Suddenly, subtle trouble becomes a major mechanical fault, still often hidden to the unskilled practitioner. These people know how to "come back" but all their efforts fail to meet their expectations. They often need help with correction of hidden mechanical dysfunction. They often become the "losers" in the health care system. Some examples might be helpful.

An old ankle injury in junior high school may be long forgotten years after college. That ankle injury might have, however, created some instability due to partial ligament tears. The ankle may have healed, full range of motion restored, and the occasional ankle sprains on the same ankle over the years long forgotten. Yet, something has changed about the way the foot hits the ground. That ankle may be just a lit-tle loose, causing slight changes in the place-ment of the foot. Repeat the place-ment of that foot on the ground thou-sands of times each day for 20 years, and soon subtle trouble may emerge as knee or low back pain.

The low back sprain or strain, or both, when it hap-pens years later, is considered a sepa-rate injury and little or no thought is given to the old ankle sprain. It may only be after years of treatment that a therapist asks about old injuries and checks the stability of the ankle. If only he/she had gotten orthotics, thinks the therapist quietly, as the foot dysfunction is seen as a faulty foundation for the low back after years of mechanical problems. But orthotics never seemed necessary, pain never a problem, until the back was injured while

Figure 25

Delayed Recovery Factors

These factors may contribute to slow recovery from a new, and seemingly minor, injury:

1. An old injury that left a joint unstable

2. An injury that left a leg length difference

3. Compensatory movement habits that have remained long after an injury has healed

4. Lack of varied recreational activities due to an old injury

5. Chronic myofascial pain syndrome from an old injury

building a deck on the back of the new dream home. The back sprain or strain cannot be shaken off, and after weeks of agony health professionals are sought. The road to recovery has many hurtles, and each one seems so atypical compared to recovery from previous injuries.

Recovery is slowed not by the actual injury sustained at the time of the soft tissue injury, but by years of strain on the back due to poor foot placement, and changes in the mechanics in the knee and hip with strain on the sacroiliac joint and low back. The pelvis may have been slightly unlevel for years without causing any problems until the back sustains injury. Muscles, overworked for years, do not recover as quickly as expected. Muscle imbalances are a problem and dis-ordered movement has only changed with the sprain or strain, not begun. An old injury has impacted a new injury, creating new and difficult problems.

A leg fracture as a child might have been a badge of honor a few days after the injury. The horseback riding might be interrupted only briefly as the weeks of casting and crutches are seen as a new and temporary means of transportation. Crutches for young kids are often a way of getting into the lunch line quickly, skipping boring gym classes and getting a bit of extra attention. The leg heals straight and quickly and the horsebacking riding is resumed. The fact that the leg is about 1/4" shorter than the other leg after the growing has been completed is not considered a problem by anyone. In fact, no one knows of its presence.

> Chronic postural problems may become a pain generator for migraine headaches, TMJ or other problems far removed from the original injury site.

A few years later, headaches turn into agonizing migraines. Since migraines are considered a vascular problem, mechanics are seldom checked for years. Instead medications are tried, often with some success and the headaches may decrease, only to return again with a new furor. No connection between the old leg fracture and leg length difference may even arise in a history intake because the migraine is seen as a vascular problem. That vascular problem needs a trigger however, and that trigger may reside in one of the muscles in the neck. When a leg length difference exists for a long time, the neck struggles to keep the head balanced and level on a foundation that is uneven. This requires a lot of work of the sternocleidomastoid muscles of the neck. These muscles harbor an uncommonly large number of TrP sites and if activated, may become a trigger for some migraine sufferers.

This sequence of migraine attacks connected to the leg length difference goes unnoticed for years.

Assessing Movement Adaptation Syndrome

Physical therapists, who might be best trained to evaluate leg length problems, are seldom involved in care for migraines. If they are, they might look at the mechanics of the entire body. They may see beyond the headache, asking the question: "Why are these symptoms present?" It is in reaching for the subtle trouble that the reward may be found. Correction of such leg length problems may require long periods of adjustment. Depending on the duration of the imbalance, the entire body has had time to adjust to muscle, ligament and other length and tension changes. Joint surfaces adjust to the imbalance. Suddenly the underlying fault is corrected, but the tissue changes need to proceed slowly. The length tension of the neck muscles must also change slowly or the migraines may return with new intensity before subsiding.

If the migraine is seen as a cascade of events which finally trigger the agonizing headache, rebalancing of the neck muscles may correct only one factor in the cascade and other factors may continue to act as triggers until alleviated. Even with perfect rebalancing the migraines may not disappear but may decrease in intensity, duration and severity. Such relief to migraine suffers is not only welcome, it is something they will fight intensely to maintain.

While only one more example follows it is easy to see that any prevous injuries can set someone up for long and painful recovery. Many of us are considered lucky to have gotten through a motor vehicle accident "without injury". I have been stopped at red lights so many times and been rear-ended that I often wonder if I would be safer going through them. Of six accidents, I have needed medical care only one time. After a few weeks that injury also healed and I returned to an active life. I have no pain, no headaches and no obvious dysfunction. But examination of muscle dysfunction reveals there is plenty of subtle trouble laying in wait if some particular kind of injury occurs.

Knowing so much about movement dysfunction I have worked to correct some of my own dysfunctions, dealing more actively with the dis-ordered movement from my lumbar fusion and years of poor mechanics. I am active, but not always pain free, if I exceed certain levels. I am more vulnerable to injuries. I make choices about what activities I am involved in, and feel lucky to be able to be so active. I also know part of that good fortune is knowing enough about movement to work hard to keep my dis-ordered movement to a minimum. I remember refusing to limp after breaking a toe several years ago, knowing that the limp would create havoc for my back. I was not willing to create problems for my back. I didn't limp and the toe settled down. When muscle havoc returns with changes in my orthotics I respect that my body needs more time to adjust than most and I try to be patient.

I want to run, to return to active hiking, but instead take slower, easier hikes and stick to biking. What should take several weeks to complete the adjustment takes twice as long; to others I may appear lazy. In my heart I am running; but I am waiting until the muscle dysfunction settles down and my potential for new injury is minimized. I have learned over the years to be patient. Some days I do better than others. But I have learned that the price I may pay for foolishness may be the creation of a long and arduous recovery. In Figure 26, muscle activity is shown using surface electromyography (sEMG) during a standard exercise. My back muscles are firing normally, reinforcing the benefits of moving with good muscle dysfunction and having less pain.

Old injuries cannot be avoided, they should not be feared. They, however, ought to be respected when subtle muscle trouble arises and returns. Such intermittent pain may be an

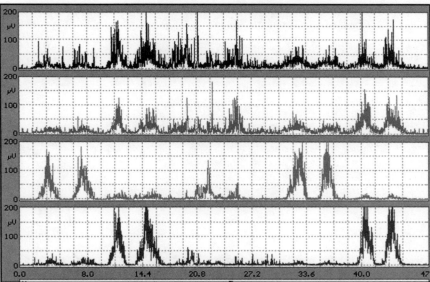

Figure 26: *The low back muscles (Chan 1&2) and the buttock muscles (Chan 3&4) are monitored during a stabilization exercise. Muscle activity is good with the expected muscles working at the correct times. In this case (the author) has had back surgery, but has retrained the muscles to fire in the expected patterns. Muscle activity changes significantly when a flare up creates pain.*

indication that other trouble lies hidden beneath the surface and self management of the symptoms before they become problems is not only wise, it is essential to continuing a healthy, active life. Lifestyle is a choice, and an active life requires a bit more maintenance as one ages. Age need not limit function, but old injuries can return to remind us we are always vulnerable to dysfunction arising from old injuries. Activity continues with aging if our choices reflect our intent to preserve an important resource, our movement patterns.

Movement Dysfunction Made Visible

The ability to use sEMG to examine muscle activity in people who are symptomatic, as shown in Figures 27 & 28 and those who are not (refer again to same exercise on previous page) allows insight into chronic pain and movement problems that has not previously been possible. Sometimes people use their muscles differently and it does not cause pain - yet. There are many questions to be answered as to when and how muscle dysfunction creates or perpetuates pain.

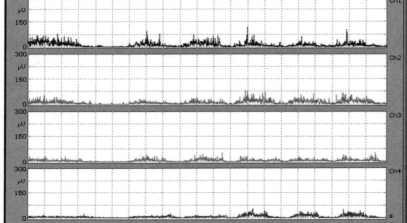

Figure 27 & 28: *These are examples of people with pain doing the same exercise as Figure 1, but who have pain. Such changes in muscle activity alters movement, often creating pain.*

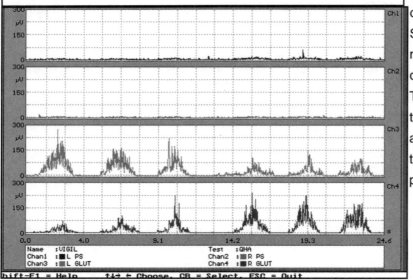

Chapter 15

Repetitive Strain Injury & Myofascial Pain Syndrome

It has been my clinical experience, that all patients with repetitive strain injury (RSI) have TrPs. My own search for understanding the profound disability of some RSI patients began with the discovery of inhibited muscles (not firing when they should) and movement dysfunction. In the most advanced cases the compensation patterns were profound. This evaluation will be described in Chapter 16.

I had learned the association between TrPs and muscle inhibition from two years of treating chronic low back pain patients before RSI patients were referred to my clinic. Just as in treating chronic low back pain problems, treating the TrPs quickly became as integral a part of the intervention for RSI. In seeking to understand why individuals doing the same job, and both developing RSI, presented with such different symptom manifestations, I began to use dynamic surface electromyography (sEMG) to explore the course of symptom development. It takes a good historian as a patient to be able to focus on what might have been symptomatic

many months before, and had been disregarded, to unravel the early signs and connect them to the symptoms at the time of the evaluation. It almost always led us to pain between the shoulder blades, even though the primary complaint was carpal tunnel syndrome or rotator cuff impingement. Loss of scapular stabilization due to overload of the stabilizing muscles and development of active TrPs became the first area assessed, regardless of presenting symptoms. From there, the course of muscle dysfunction took one of several routes. Several of the RSI syndromes are described in Figure 29.

Why one RSI syndrome rather than another evolves can be a matter only of conjecture. Factors which may play a role are, even at first glance, too numerous to measure. The presence of one or more of these factors may have an impact on symptoms that develop in one individual as compared to another.

What became the greatest complaint that I had difficulty understanding was the fatigue at carrying out the simplest tasks, including physi-

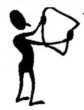

Figure 29

Common Syndromes Related to RSI

1. Carpal Tunnel Syndrome: This tunnel is designed to protect the nerves and vessels entering the hand. Bones form three sides, a tough ligament the roof of the tunnel.

2. Shoulder Impingement Syndrome: This problem results from poor scapular stabilization, or damage to the rotator cuff, i.e., the ligaments and muscle attachments around the shoulder. Changes in how the shoulder moves may result in clicking, popping, or painful arcs in the range.

3. Headaches: When TrPs develop in certain muscles in the upper back, neck and shoulders, referred pain patterns cause a number of headache complaints.

4. Lateral Epicondylitis: This inflammation (often referred to as "tennis elbow") may result from minute tears of the tendon where it attaches on the bone, chronic inflammation, &/or TrPs.

5. DeQuervain's: This is an inflammation of the tendon at the base of the thumb. Acute pain is felt at the thumb side of the wrist.

6. Thoracic Outlet Syndrome: This involves the muscles at the neck and shoulder blades, with changes in posture, TrPs and shortening of muscles. Compression of the nerves and vessels as they go into the arm contribute to a variety of RSI complaints, including carpal tunnel syndrome.

7. Focal Dystonia (Writer's Cramp): This condition is an involuntary cramping of the hand and can become quite severe.

Any and all of these problems require a careful diagnosis from a health care professional familiar with RSI. Symptoms can present as other problems.

Refer to Appendix C for References/Recommended Reading

cal demands therapists had once categorized as "light duty." Again, the sEMG measures provided clues. The rapid fatigue I saw and the profoundly slow recovery was what I found defined the length of treatment and the interventions chosen.

Treatment

For RSI patients, treatment begins with treatment of the TrPs. The TrPs seemed the initial factor in the development of muscle inhibition. I sought to reverse the process from its beginning much as I had done with low back pain patients. Fortunately for me, it was at about this time that Dr. Simons entered my world, offering me a depth of knowledge about TrPs I could only otherwise have gained at a snail's pace.

Following the deactivation/ treatment of the TrPs, I had to get the muscle working again. This new challenge took a level of creativity I had never experienced in

25 years as a physical therapist. Without sEMG I would never have stayed on course. What I learned shook the very foundation of my physical therapy training and a new paradigm emerged. Patients could not simply "make the muscle work" no matter how hard they tried. They could not make the connection between the brain and the muscle that should have responded to the brain's commands.

Once the muscle was working it was still very vulnerable. Just 2-3 repetitions with resistance would often shut the muscle down, the TrP once again active. I was moving through a maze or puzzle, and sEMG my primary guide.

What was fascinating was that resolution of symptoms in the hand could be accomplished by deactivation of the TrPs in the neck and shoulder. Finding the source became the prize I cherished most. The lack of scapular stabilization in the RSI patients was

Figure 30

Factors Determining RSI Symptom Presentation

1. Old injuries

2. Posture

3. Structural asymmetry

4. Specifics of task performance between individuals

5. Age

6. Muscle length, tone, play between muscles

7. Medical problems, i.e., diabetes, arthritis

8. Motor control adaptation

9. Genetic predisposition

profound. Simple exercise would inhibit muscle activity for hours. Sitting at a keyboard, typing with an improper technique became the common villian. Long, low level physical demands on these muscles was what had to be changed. The fatigue and failure to recover was the predictor of treatment length and outcome.

Avoiding Surgery

Patients scheduled for carpal tunnel surgery could often resolve their symptoms by correction of proximal biomechanics and myofascial TrPs. Impingement syndromes of the shoulders often likewise resolved. Tennis elbow, resistant to all treatment, resolved with correction of scapular and shoulder dysfunction. At the bottom of all these movement dsyfunctions were TrPs. Myofascial pain syndrome was no longer a problem primarily of referred muscle pain but of muscle and movement dysfunction. For TrPs to remain deactivated, perpetuating factors need to be found and resolved.

In the case of patients with rotator cuff damage for whom surgery was recommended, I found that correction of the mechanics of how the shoulder moved was often sufficient to eliminate symptoms and allow adequate return of function. However the problem manifests itself, close examination of the precipitating factors triggering the development of the symptoms might lead to non-surgical resolution.

It is often the case that following successful carpal tunnel surgery the symptoms return. Often the proximal symptoms become worse. This may not mean that the carpal tunnel surgery was unnecessary, only that the other symptoms also need to be treated, and the biomechanical problems of movement addressed. Otherwise, treatment of the primary complaint, i.e., the carpal tunnel, may not result in the long term and permanent functional and symptom changes expected.

RSI in the Work Place

The increased understanding of RSI has lead to increased interest in prevention of RSI problems at the worksite. Often this requires examination of how the employee is interacting with their workstation. Work station ergonomic design has come a long way, and many changes have been implemented into companies who have seen some reduction in RSI problems, but not what was expected. The next step is to examine how the user, the employee, is interfacing with the work station. It is not uncommon to find simple movement patterns that have become habits and interfere with good movement mechanics at a workstation. This cannot always be visually discovered. The use of sEMG at the worksite can be very valuable.

Teaching employees the interaction

between their level of stress, fatigue or frustration and the muscle activity in performing their jobs can have a very positive impact on muscle activity. Small habits and changes in worksite items can have large changes in the work load on a muscle. How one approaches using a mouse, and how one takes best advantage of short breaks in work tasks can significantly impact the fatigue level of muscles at the end of the workday.

Examination of employees before they develop symptoms, educating them into self management techniques such as the ones described in this book and teaching them proactive techniques to change the factors leading to RSI, can make a big change in employee problems. RSI interferes with everything that someone does. There is a sense of hopelessness and helplessness that comes with advanced RSI, when the medical community offers so little, that makes it imperative that everyone make prevention their primary target for this syndrome.

Chapter 16

When Movement Hurts. Examination with Surface Electromyography

Movement is a complex task. Smooth, efficient movement may be likened to a symphony orchestra. Each instrument must be in tune and each instrument must play its part (and only its part) at the proper time. If the violins are on page one and the trumpets, flutes, and percussion are on page three the music will be "out of synch" and not sound as intended. So to, the muscles must perform when they should (and only when they should) in harmony with the other muscles needed for movement. Without the proper orchestration of muscles, the various joint movements will not occur with the proper timing.

If we had to consciously call to action each muscle, and consciously determine how fast and how powerful each muscle must be to complete a specific task, such simple actions as drinking a cup of coffee or brushing our teeth would suddenly be very complex, slow and energy consuming. For the young child learning to walk, they must fall many times before the

proper muscle sequence becomes automatic. With the ability to perform a task without prolonged conscious effort, a motor plan is completed.

Motor plans allow us to perform many tasks without conscious effort and energy. The body seeks inherently to compile a motor plan that is efficient. It is the efficiency and effortlessness of a well rehearsed movement plan that produces the grace we so admire in the elite gymnist or ballet dancer.

Injury

When any animal is injured we see an immediate change in movement patterns. There is an attempt to protect the area from further injury. The change in motor plan may be a limp, a stiffened gait or a limitation of range of motion. If the protective movement is needed for any length of time, it too becomes a motor plan. This compensatory motor plan serves a necessary function until the original injury is healed.

The problem often arises when the injury has healed and the compensatory motor plan remains the habituated movement of choice. Over time, the compensatory motor plan begins to cause pain. The perpetuating factor in pain is the compensatory motor plan which is often using the 'wrong' muscles to accomplish the task. The muscles that are primarily responsible for performing the task are not working, the "second string" muscles pinch hit and continue to function. They are less efficient and place biomechanical stresses on the joint and soft tissue. Over time, injury may develop in these muscles, further spreading and perpetuating the pain.

Assessment

The goal in assessing movement dysfunction is that these compensatory motor plans can be identified and changed. Restoring healthy, normal motor plans will increase efficiency and decrease stress to muscles, joints and soft tissue. While not all muscles can be assessed without invasive techniques, sEMG measurement offers unique insight into the movement dysfunction.

Using sEMG sensors which stick like bandaids to the skin, placed strategically over certain muscles, a picture can be drawn of any movement dysfunction that may be contributing to pain and decreased function.

Such an assessment must include numerous muscles to obtain an accurate profile. The assessment must also include a wide variety of movement patterns, as dysfunction may occur in only a few movement patterns. The ability to execute and interpret the assessment requires someone highly trained in this technique.

Case Study

A brief look at a sEMG profile for movement adaptation syndrome may help you understand how the evaluation can focus treatment planning and facilitate the desired outcome.

This patient was a 32 year old female who was injured while working as a housekeeper. She had symptoms in her right hand, neck and left elbow. Six months after the injury she underwent surgery of the right arm and hand for carpal tunnel syndrome, along with a release of a nerve in her arm. The right hand numbness and right elbow pain were better after surgery. She could lift her arm a bit better and she could make a tight fist.

What had not improved was pain in the upper arm, a sense of fatigue and difficulty lifting things using that arm. Her shoulder range of motion felt like it was "blocked" and indeed she had painful limited range of the shoulder in full flexion, abduction, extension and external rotation. She found writing difficult and painful, and described her fingers as "clumsy, not working right" when she tried to pick things up. She had not had any therapy for TrPs prior to being seen for the sEMG evaluation.

Examination of her posture revealed that she was not holding the right shoulder blade in the same location as the left. Both shoulders were more rounded and forward than the normal alignment. Multiple trigger points were found in the anterior deltoid, supraspinatus, infraspinatus, lower trapezius and subscapularis.

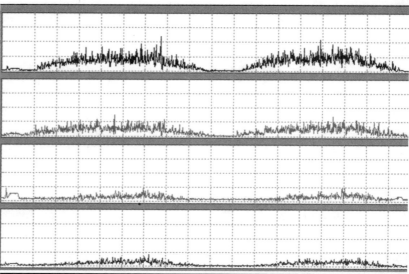

Figure 31: *Four shoulder muscles: 1) Anterior deltoid; 2) Supraspinatus; 3) Infraspinatus; 4) Lower trapezius are monitored during resisted shoulder flexion. Channel 1 (top) and Channel 2 (bottom) should show much more activity. Such changes in muscle activity can result in pain & movement dysfunction. In this case the result was a funtional shoulder impingement.*

Surgery had been recommended for her shoulder. It was felt that repair of the tear in her cuff and removal of a small calcium deposit would be necessary for her to have any symptom relief and increase in function. Prior to authorizing surgery the patient was sent for a sEMG evaluation and treatment as indicated.

The sEMG evaluation demonstrated that she had poor stabilization of her shoulder blade. Along with dysfunction in a rotator cuff muscle, the cup portion of the shoulder joint was malpositioned when the arm was moved.

The head of the humerus was, therefore, malpositioned in the socket as the arm was moved upward. This caused the arm to get "blocked" and feel "stuck".

To simplify her sEMG data, comparisons have been made between her initial evaluation and her discharge evaluation with data that have come from only one of the many dynamic functional tests done. The activity is the same pre and post treatment for comparison. The patterns of how the muscles are firing are more important that the exact amplitude of any one muscle. Certain muscles are expected

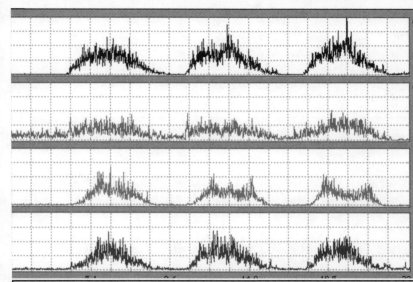

Figure 32: *Four shoulder muscles: 1) Anterior deltoid; 2) Supraspinatus; 3) Infraspinatus; 4) Lower trapezius are monitored during resisted shoulder flexion after treatment. There is much better stabilization of the shoulder blade (bottom) and higher activity from the prime mover (top). This corrects movement dysfunction within the joint & reduces pain.*

self, and to reinforce the problem solving nature of her home program. She was also given a stretching program and asked to complete the stretches when the TrPs had been worked on.

Because her fatigue in the muscles expected to stabilize the shoulder blade was so signficant, exercise was added slowly and carefully using the sEMG equipment to measure changes in fatigue and assist in designing changes to the program. When one goal was reached, another was set.

to work during each task and certain muscles are expected to do less or to be silent. In examining these data, comparisons are made between how the muscles behave actively and how they work when weight or loading is added to the task. In this patient, when the demand increased by adding resistance, the muscles worked less. This is often an indication that active trigger points are present. This muscle inhibition tends to increase the compensatory movement problems when any strengthening program is attempted.

Treatment consisted of teaching the patient how to work on the trigger points her-

Changes could be documented with the sEMG before she began to feel better. This is often the case when an active TrP is interfering with function and pain. Several sessions were needed to deactivate the subscapularis TrP, one she could not reach herself, as it lies hidden under the shoulder blade. With treatment of this TrP she began to feel better and was more willing to move her arm. She began each session showing off what she could do that was not possible the week before. Changes came more rapidly and she could begin some gentle strengthening.

Surgery was avoided with 12 sessions of treatment. She had some minimal permanent restrictions to protect the tear in her rotator cuff, but these did not affect daily function. She had little pain unless she overdid it. If this happened she knew which TrPs to go after. Perhaps most important, she felt she had some control over the pain. She had become her own symptom manager.

Case of the Sore Thumb

Many different kinds of movement adaptation syndrome (MAS) can be examined with sEMG. In the following example, a therapist does manual therapy several days a week and otherwise spends hours at a computer doing word processing and graphics develops a very localized complaint of pain at the base of the thumb. After ruling out carpal tunnel syndrome, a sEMG evaluation was done to determine if muscle function was within expected ranges.

Treatment will include not only reduction of the tendinitis but reactivation of the opponens muscle in the hand. If this is not part of the program the tendinitis may recur when activity is increased.

In this person, proximal muscle dysfunction does exist and is also being addressed.

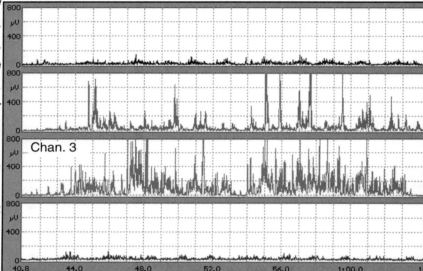

Figure 33: *The critical muscle during the task of pinching clothespins is the small thumb muscle. The left thumb muscle (channel 3) is working well in this hand. Other muscles on this graph are not critical.*

Changes made in typing schedule and modifications to how physical demands are performed, as well as manual therapy have also be helpful in symptom reduction. A history of multiple motor vehicle accidents may also be a factor in increasing the vulnerability of someone to other injuries or dysfunction. Staying healthy is a commitment in maintaining good movement and balance skills as well as in choices about eating, stress management and exercise.

MAS Evaluations

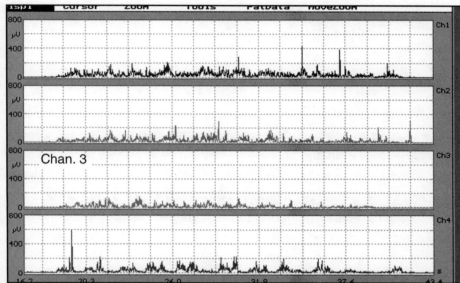

Figure 34: *In this same test, the painful side shows almost no activity in the right thumb muscle (channel 3).*

ronment can make significant changes in symptoms.

When the working environment is considered to be the major contributing factor in the perpetuation of myofascial pain syndrome or movement dysfunction, an analysis of the employee interacting with their workstation can evaluate a number of physiologic risk factors. This is particularly important in repetitive strain injury where the static or repetitive task must be changed in some way.

Many physical and some occupational therapists can perform an abbreviated version of this assessment with smaller, more portable equipment. The more chronic and complex your symptoms, the more you might benefit from a full evaluation. Such an evaluation must include consideration of postural problems, both structural and functional. Many perpetuating factors need to be considered, including dietary, biomechanics, chronic stress and limb proportions. Often simple changes in the envi-

195

Chapter 17

Self-Help Techniques

There are several techniques that have been mentioned on preceding pages. These techniques may be best performed with the assistance of a therapist skilled in the techniques, but many of them can be performed by you with a little practice. Patients with more complex and chronic problems will find these techniques may aggravate their symptoms and they should not be attempted without assistance.

Four techniques will be described briefly. Some of the techniques are more general than others which have specific applications.

Contract-Relax

This technique often helps a tight muscle to relax and lengthen, thus providing greater stretch to a tight band. The technique is based on the principle that following a strong contraction there is a strong relaxation.

The muscle is taken to a comfortable point near its tight end range. Shortening of the

muscle is prohibited, while the muscle contracts. This isometric contraction is held for about three seconds. As the muscle relaxes there is a passive attempt to stretch the muscle or add to its lengthening. Any increase in length is where the muscle next is held for another isometric contraction. After the contraction, relaxation is followed by an attempt to increase the passive lengthening.

This contract-relax technique is repeat-

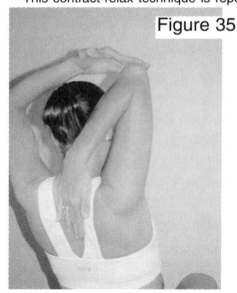

Figure 35

ed 3-5 times after which the stretch may be held for 20-30 seconds. The contraction need not be the strongest possible; a moderate, careful contraction is sufficient. The contraction should not be so quick that it is very painful, as this may increase the muscle dysfunction.

Hair Pulling

This technique has been very beneficial for individuals with headaches and TMJ pain, especially those involved in motor vehicle accidents. Under the scalp there are several layers of tissue that slide over the skull. Even without impact of the head hitting glass or other structures in the car, there develop areas of the scalp that seem to get "stuck" to the skull. These areas often become significant pain generators. The ability of the tissues to slide must be restored.

The entire scalp should be examined to determine where the tightness is located. These areas may be too sensitive to treat directly right away. More indirect techniques may be used initially to make the area less sensitive. See the last paragraph of this section for recommendations.

To perform this technique loosely grasp the hair and make a gradual fist. As the first becomes tighter there will be an increase in tension on the scalp. The person should feel a release in 10-15 seconds if the scalp technique

is working. The fist can then be tightened a fraction more. If another release can be achieved tighten the fist again. As this technique pro-

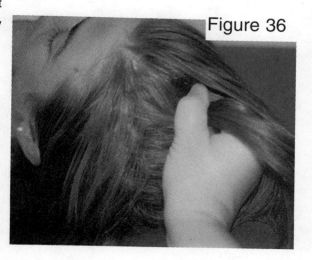

Figure 36

gresses the releases should come more quickly. Tension may be increased by rotating the scalp slightly.

If the technique rapidly evokes a headache the technique may be preceeded by using a vibrator to make the area less sensitive. A very flexible attachment must be used initially, and the most sensitive areas should be covered rapidly. Painful areas can be easily identified as generating symptoms. Areas may take several weeks to desensitize before techniques such as hair pulling can be tolerated.

Stripping Massage

This technique involves a long, deep

pressure along the length of the muscle belly. The movement generally goes from distal to proximal (toward the direction of the center of the body) and is slow, even in pressure, and firm. This type of massage cannot be tolerated by many individuals initially and must be developed slowly without increased pain. The rollers on the TAMM Unit or Intracell may be helpful in developing a tolerance to this technique. Pressure can be added gradually as tolerated.

The stripping massage can be done along the length of the taut band, with or without a massage oil or lotion. More friction may

Figure 37

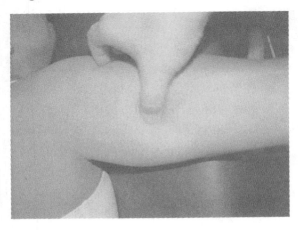

be desirable in some individuals or may be increased over time as the muscle becomes less painful.

Stripping massage often leaves a soreness afterwards that should not be excessive,

i.e., should not last more than 2-3 hours. The discomfort should be different from the normal symptoms and should feel only like a slight bruising. This should resolve within a few hours unless the massage was too forceful. Drinking plenty of water after the massage is helpful.

Cross Fiber Technique

The use of cross fiber or transverse friction techniques is often most helpful when the musculotendinous junction (MTJ) or attachment of the muscle to the bone is painful. This represents some form of overuse strain of the tissue in this area, possibly due to the shortening in the area of the taut band and TrP. The transverse massage is performed initially with a light pressure, to be increased after 1-2 minutes as the tenderness subsides. Often the massage reduces the pain considerably and pressure can be increased. If pain increases, too much pressure may have been used. Try later, using less pressure to start. After 3-4 minutes the pressure should be deep enough to increase the motion of the deeper tissues for which this technique is used.

This technique is initially often very painful and a health care provider should demonstrate the technique before it is done as a self management tool. Treatment should result in an increase in painless ROM. It should provide several hours of relief. Care should be taken to not rub the skin back and forth, creating a blister. Without lotion, the skin should move with the finger. Ice can be used after the treatment to reduce post-treatment soreness.

Exhalation

The careful use of deep breathing and relaxing while putting a stretch on the involved muscle may also be helpful. The initial pressure on the TrP is often painful. By carefully taking a deep breath and relaxing, a stretch can be applied at the same time as the exhalation, allowing the muscle to lengthen.

Additional pressure may be applied with the pressure tool at the same time that a slow exhalation, or letting go of the breath, is performed. There is greater relaxation of the muscle at that time, and gentle stretch is also better tolerated.

Appendix A

Range of Motion Planes

The range of motion (ROM)planes are important in understanding how to do the exercises correctly. They are somewhat difficult to present in two dimensions, and you are encouraged to refer to the <u>Anatomy of Movemen</u>t reference in Appendix C.

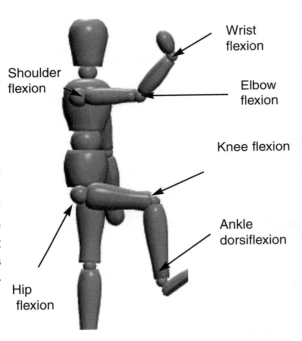

Flexion-Extension

Flexion and extension occur in what is called the sagital plane. This plane, in mid-line, divides the body into right and left sides. The flexion-extension movement occurs parallel to that line. Movement of the various joints cannot be defined by a simple rule, so the model has been marked with as many movements as possible.

- Flexion of the head and trunk would be movement toward the fetal position.
- Making a fist and curling the toes down are flexion.
- Walking on heels dorsiflexes the ankle.
- Walking on toes plantarflexes the ankle.
- Bending the ear down to touch the shoulder is lateral flexion.

Abduction-Adduction

The frontal plane, in mid-line, would cut the body into a front half and back half. Extending this line provides the plane for abduction and adduction. *Abduction* is generally away from the body, *adduction* toward the midline of the body.

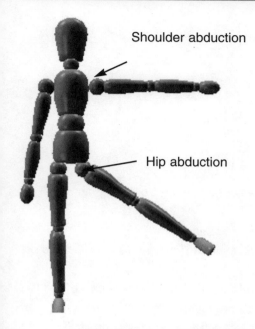

Shoulder abduction

Hip abduction

a top and bottom half. When the rotation occurs with movement away from the midline, it is external rotation, Internal rotation refers to rotation into the center.

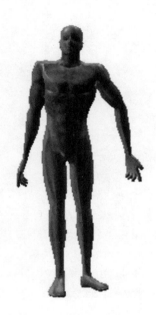

Making angels in the snow is a good example of abduction-adduction.

- Spreading the fingers apart would be abduction, closing them would be adduction.
- Scapular adduction is generally called retraction, and scapular abduction referred to as protraction.
- The foot motion is called eversion (turning the foot out, as if you wanted only to walk on the inside edge of the foot) and inversion (turning the foot in, so only the outer edge of the foot would touch the ground).

- Turning the entire leg so the toes point out to the side is external rotation (of the hip).
- Turning the palms from the normal inward position so they face out is external rotation of the shoulder and supination of the forearm.

Rotation

Rotation of the body occurs around the transverse plane which would cut the body into

Appendix B

Abbreviations & Glossary

Abbreviations

CTD	Cumulative trauma disorder
CTS	Carpal tunnel syndrome
LTR	Lower trapezius
MAS	Movement adaptation syndrome
MPS	Myofascial pain syndrome
MVA	Motor vehicle accident
ROM	Range of motion
RSI	Repetitive strain injury
SCM	Sternocleidomastoid
TFL	Tensor fascia latae
TMD	Temporomandibular disease
TMJ	Temporomandibular joint
TOS	Thoracic outlet syndrome
TrPs	Trigger points
UTR	Upper trapezius

Glossary

Active TrP: a TrP within a taut band which is painful when pressure is applied to it and which refers pain or symptoms that the indi-vidual recognizes as part of their pain com-plaint

Angina: chest pain

Anterior: facing toward the front or located on the front

Autonomic dysfunction: when part of the autonomic nervous system is not working prop-erly, as in someone being very sensitive to light touch

Axillary: in the region under the arm; armpit

Bruxism: grinding of the teeth

Bursitis: inflammation of a bursa, or sac locat-ed to reduce friction between tissues

Carpal tunnel syndrome: when the median nerve is pinched, or compressed, as it goes through a "tunnel" at the wrist, under a tight lig-ament

Cervical: neck portion of spine

Concentric contraction: when the muscle shortens as it contracts

Deactivate: make TrP less sensitive; active TrP becomes latent

Deep: underneath other muscles or structures, closer to the inside of the body

Disc disease: discs are the shock absorbers

between each bone in the spinal column

Distal: further from the center, as opposed to proximal

Dysfunction: abnormal or impaired function, such as muscles working incorrectly

Eccentric contraction: when the muscle lengthens as it contracts, such as when the biceps contracts as the arm lowers a heavy book to the table

Entrapment: when one tissue, such as a nerve, is caught in other tissue

Epicondylitis: inflammation at the elbow

Exaccerbate: to aggravate or make worse

Fibromyalgia: painful, chronic widespread musculoskeletal pain, often with rapid muscle fatigue, non-refreshing sleep and tender points

Flaccid: hanging loose or limp

Frozen shoulder: a term referring to pain and inability to move the shoulder and/or the shoulder blade

Medial: closer to the midline of the body

Hypermobile: with more motion in the joint than normal or expected

Hypomobile: with less motion in the joint than expected; decreased ROM

Idiopathic: when the cause of the problem is unknown

Immobilization: to prevent movement of a joint or limb

Latent TrP: a TrP in a taut band that causes pain when pressure is applied, but which does not contribute to the primary referral of pain

Lateral: further from the midline of the body

Lumbar: low back region

Malocculusion: when the top and bottom teeth meet incorrectly

Movement adaptation syndrome: when pain and muscle dysfunction results in changes from the normal way of moving, becoming a habit and often becoming the cause of pain, rather than the result over time

Myalgia: pain in muscle

Myopain: pain in muscle

Orthotics: a specially fit device designed to activate, support or correct the position or alignment of a joint or joints, e.g., orthotics to correct foot positioning

Overuse: when the same movement is repeated for hours or one position is held for long periods of time, resulting in strain on tissue that does not occur when a variety of movement is done

Pain generator: tissue (i.e., muscle, ligament) from which the pain arises

Pinched nerve: when a nerve root is compressed by tissue, i.e., it exits from the spine

Posterior: facing toward or located at the back side

Postlaminectomy: after surgery to the spine where portions of the disc and vertebra are removed

Postural asymmetry: refers to posture that is not balanced, i.e., one shoulder is higher than the other

Prone: lying face downward

Pronation: turning the hand so the palm faces

down or back

Proximal: closer to the center, as opposed to distal

Rotator cuff: the capsule around the shoulder joint

Scapula: the shoulder blade

Scoliosis: curvature of the spine from side to side

Shin splints: painful strain of muscles on the anterior (front) surface of the lower leg, often from running on hard surfaces

Spondylosis: any of various degenerative diseases of the spine

Stabilizers: when muscles are used to stabilize or hold one part of the body so that another can work more efficiently, e.g., when muscles stabilize the shoulder blade so that the arm can move more efficiently

Subluxation: looseness of a joint, often from a tear in the capsule surrounding the joint

Superficial: on or near the outside or near the surface of the body

Supination: turning the palm face up or forward facing

Supine: lying face up

Temporomandibular: joint on both sides of jaw; opens and closes mouth

Temporomandibular disease: when changes occur in and around the TMJ

Tendonitis: inflammation of the tendon

Thoracic: chest portion of spine

Thoracic outlet syndrome:

Tinnitus: ringing in the ears

Vertigo: dizziness, the sense that one has of having the surroundings whirling about

Whiplash: rapid flexion and extension of neck, as occurs in MVA or fall

Winging: when the medial border of the scapula (close to the spine) protrudes more than normal

Appendix C

References, Product Information

References

Cailliet R: <u>Soft Tissue Pain and Disability</u>. Philadelphia: F.A.Davis Co. 1986

Headley BJ: Physiologic Risk Factors, in Sanders M (ed) <u>Management of Cumulative Trauma Disorders</u>, Butterworth-Heinemann, Scheduled publication early 1997.

Headley BJ: Chronic pain management. in O'Sullivan SB & Schmitz TJ (eds) <u>Physical Rehabilitation: Assessment and Treatment</u> (2nd Ed), Philadelphia: FA Davis Co., 1988
Mense, S: Nociception from skeletal muscle in relation to clinical muscle pain. Pain, 54:241-289, 1993.

Leyzer RB: <u>Muscle Pain, Cramps and Fatigue</u>, Chap 67. In AG Engel, C. Franzini-Armstrong, Myology, Ed.2, Vol. 2, McGraw-Hill, New York, 1994

Mense S, Simons DG: <u>Muscle Pain: Understanding its nature, diagnosis and treatment</u>. Williams & Willkins, Baltimore (Scheduled publication 1997)

Russell IJ: Neurochemical pathogenesis of fibromyalgia syndrome. J Musculoskeletal Pain 4:61-92, 1996

Simons DG: Referred phenomena of myofascial trigger points. in Vecchiet L et al (eds) <u>New Trends in Referred Pain and Hyperalgesia</u>. Elsevier Science Pub, 1993.

Travel, JG, Simons DG: <u>Myofascial Pain and Dysfunction. The Trigger Point Manual. Vol. 1 The Upper Extremities</u>. Baltimore:Williams & Wilkins, 1983.

Travell JG, Simons DG: <u>Myofascial Pain and Dysfunction. The Trigger Point Manual. Vol 2. The Lower Extremities</u>. Baltimore: Williams & Wilkins, 1992.

Recommended Reading

Calais-Germain B: <u>Anatomy of Movement</u>. Seattle: Eastland Press.1993

Starlanyl D, Copeland ME:<u> Fibromyalgia & Chronic Myofascial Pain Syndrome. A Survival Manual</u>. Oakland CA: New Harbinger Publications, Inc. 1996

Pascarelli E, Quilter D: <u>Repetitive Strain Injury. A Computer User's Guide</u>. New York: John Wiley & Sons, Inc. 1994.

Product Information

OPTP
P.O. Box 47009
Minneapolis MN 55447
800/367-7393   or 612/553-0452

Patient & Professional Catelogs
TheraCane
IntraCell
TAMM Unit
Disc-O-Sit

Index

Notes

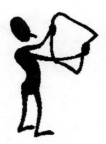

It is through adversity that we learn the skills needed to reach our dreams

-bj's soul scraps